186

Plain X-ray Diagnosis of the Acute Abdomen

Plain X-ray Diagnosis of the Acute Abdomen

A Surgical Handbook with Notes on Clinical Presentation and Differential Diagnosis

MALCOLM H. GOUGH MS(Lond), FRCS(Eng)
Surgeon, The John Radcliffe Hospital, Oxford

MICHAEL W.L. GEAR DM, MCh(Oxon), FRCS(Eng)
Surgeon, Gloucestershire Royal Hospital

ABDALLAH S. DAAR DPhil(Oxon), MRCP, FRCS(Eng & Ed)
Surgeon and Director of Transplant Unit,
Mafraq Hospital, Abu Dhabi, United Arab Emirates

SECOND EDITION

BLACKWELL SCIENTIFIC PUBLICATIONS

OXFORD LONDON EDINBURGH

BOSTON PALO ALTO MELBOURNE

Editorial offices:
Osney Mead, Oxford, OX2 0EL
8 John Street, London, WC1N 2ES
23 Ainslie Place, Edinburgh, EH3 6AJ
52 Beacon Street, Boston
Massachusetts 02108, USA
667 Lytton Avenue, Palo Alto
California 94301, USA
107 Barry Street, Carlton
Victoria 3053, Australia

First published 1971
Second edition 1986

Photoset by Enset (Photosetting)
Midsomer Norton, Bath, Avon
and printed and bound
in Great Britain by

Printed and bound in Great Britain by
William Clowes Limited, Beccles and London

DISTRIBUTORS

USA
Blackwell Mosby Book Distributors
11830 Westline Industrial Drive
St Louis, Missouri 63141

Canada
The C.V. Mosby Company
5240 Finch Avenue East,
Scarborough, Ontario

Australia
Blackwell Scientific Publications
(Australia) Pty Ltd
107 Barry Street, Carlton
Victoria 3053

British Library
Cataloguing in Publication Data

Gough, Malcolm H.
Plain X-ray diagnosis of the acute abdomen: a surgical handbook with notes on clinical presentation and differential diagnosis.—2nd ed.
1. Abdomen—Radiography
I. Title II. Gear, Michael W.L. III. Daar, Abdallah S.
617.550757 RC944

ISBN 0-632-01432-6

Contents

Preface

Taken in conjunction with a history and clinical examination the plain X-ray film may provide invaluable help in reaching or confirming a diagnosis in the patient presenting with an acute abdomen.

This book has been designed as a practical guide to the interpretation of the plain abdominal X-ray. We hope that the casualty officer or trainee surgeon, who usually has to make the initial assessment of the X-ray, will find it useful and that the addition of possible alternative diagnoses suggested by the X-ray will enhance its value.

Radiology as a speciality has undergone considerable advance since the first edition of the book was published in 1971. Most hospitals have better X-ray departments, and ultrasonography, computerized tomography and isotope scanning have all contributed to an improvement in patient care. Recent radiological text books often include chapters on the interpretation of the plain abdominal X-ray but these have generally been written with the radiologist in mind. We think that there continues to be a need for an easily read account for the junior surgeon of the value and potential of the plain abdominal X-ray in the diagnosis of the 'acute abdomen'.

The radiographs discussed in the first edition were carefully selected and although some have been replaced and many added we have found little reason for major change in the overall format of the book. The additions were required because there were some important omissions, e.g. mesenteric infarction, hiatus hernia and intestinal pseudo obstruction. Fifteen years ago necrotizing enterocolitis was hardly recognized as a clinical entity: it has since become one of the commoner causes of the acute abdomen in the neonatal period. The addition of this condition is part of a larger review of the whole section on paediatric diseases.

Representative X-ray films have been grouped in chapters under the headings: Alimentary System; Genito-urinary System; Trauma; Infancy and Childhood; and Miscellaneous Opacities. The legend accompanying each film has been divided, where appropriate, into four sections:

1 The characteristic radiological signs demonstrated in the film.
2 The differential diagnosis suggested by the X-ray.

In order to make the account of greater value to the clinician—for this is designed as a clinical, not a radiological handbook—we have included:

3 an account of the common presenting symptoms and signs of the condition under discussion; and
4 a list of possible clinical differential diagnoses.

We have recognized that it is difficult to produce a complete differential diagnosis in each instance without making the list unwieldy. Our aim has been to suggest common alternative diagnoses; reference may then be made to other films and legends in the book.

We have not discussed the use of contrast media, for example barium studies or arteriography, or other investigations such as ultrasonography or computerized axial tomography because these investigations require the presence of a radiologist. However, a note is frequently made in the text whenever one of these special techniques might be indicated.

The varying penetration by X-rays

of bone, soft tissues and gas provides sufficient contrast for diagnosis in most acute abdominal conditions. The size, shape and position of such viscera as the liver, spleen and kidneys are often identifiable on the X-ray as shadows of varying density, as are abnormal masses such as abscesses or aneurysms. The familiar black translucency (transradiancy) of gas outlines the bowel in its normal or pathological state and may also be present in abnormal sites following a perforation or laparotomy.

A normal amount of extraperitoneal fat may be helpful in delineating the lateral margins of the peritoneal cavity (the 'flank stripe'); an excess of abdominal fat, ascitic fluid or an adjacent inflammatory process may obscure this and other detail. In some patients with an acute abdomen X-rays will be unnecessary or inadvisable. There is little need further to investigate obvious acute appendicitis, and in some conditions, for example ruptured ectopic pregnancy, delay in operation may be harmful. In other seriously ill patients X-ray examination may be most helpful. As well as establishing or confirming the diagnosis additional information, often of an unexpected nature, may be obtained. However, **if clinical signs indicate that operation is necessary negative or equivocal X-ray findings should be ignored.** The investigation may be carried out without delaying surgery during the period of pre-operative resuscitation. It should be performed in the X-ray Department as portable machines often do not produce satisfactory resolution. If an automatic processing machine is not available, films should be allowed to dry: wet films are not as easy to interpret owing to the refractive effect of water.

A radiograph of the chest should usually be performed as well as the abdominal films as intrathoracic disease may produce pain which is referred to the abdomen. In addition conditions unrelated to the pain but relevant to the management of the patient, and especially to the administration of an anaesthetic may be revealed, e.g. cardiac or aortic enlargement, carcinoma of the lung, pulmonary tuberculosis.

When a patient is ill and in pain it is important to reduce the discomfort of any diagnostic procedure as much as possible. If, on admission to the hospital, the patient is placed on a trolley having a radiolucent top which can be positioned over a pedestal Bucky, X-rays may be taken with the minimum of disturbance. The usual plain X-ray is taken with the patient in the supine position but occasionally a prone view may provide different information, e.g. in the supine view gastric air outlines the antrum and part of the body of the stomach, while in the prone view it outlines the fundus.

Films are also frequently taken in the erect posture in order to demonstrate free gas, or gas-fluid levels in the intestine. If this might cause severe discomfort to the patient, or even produce hypotensive effects, 'side up' films with the patient lying alternately on the left or right side with a horizontal X-ray beam are preferable, and give as good or even better information. In this lateral decubitus position gas will flow from one side of a viscus to the other and may, for example, more accurately indicate the site of an obstruction. Time must be allowed for this shift of gas to occur before the film is taken. A lateral erect film may be required to localize an opacity seen on the supine or antero-posterior erect view in order to differentiate, for example, a renal from a gallbladder calculus or to confirm calcification in an abdominal aortic aneurysm.

Chapter 1
Introduction

HOW TO USE THIS BOOK

If confirmation of a provisional diagnosis is sought, refer to this diagnosis in the Index. This will allow comparison of the patient's X-ray films with typical examples. Each example has a list of alternative radiological and clinical disgnoses.

If the diagnosis is in doubt, the films should be examined carefully and systematically as described below. Appearances considered to be abnormal should be checked by referring to the appropriate radiological sign in the index. This will enable a typical example of the condition to be studied and the accompanying text will provide a differential diagnosis.

X-rays of conditions specifically occurring in infancy and childhood are, for ease of reference, considered separately in Chapter 5.

EXAMINATION OF AN ABDOMINAL X-RAY FILM

Many will have evolved their own system of examination but one method is outlined below.

A knowledge of normal appearance and common variations is necessary before the significance of a particular X-ray feature can be assessed (Figs 1–4). Each film must be systematically examined. It should be emphasized that only if the quality of the film is good can reliable information be obtained. A viewing box should always be used.

The temptation to note only the most obvious abnormality and to make a snap diagnosis must be resisted.

It should be noted that it is conventional to view X-ray films as if one were facing the patient. Thus, 'right side' refers to the patient's right and not to the right side of the film. This convention is followed throughout the book.

The patients name, the date of the X-ray and the accuracy of the right and left labelling should be checked on all X-rays.

THE SYSTEMATIC EXAMINATION OF A PLAIN X-RAY FILM OF THE ABDOMEN

1. Bones

Joint and disc spaces
Cortical outlines
Trabecular pattern
Density of bones generally
Areas of lysis or sclerosis
Fractures
Epiphyseal lines if present

2. Soft tissue shadows

Normal viscera
Abdominal wall:
  diaphragm
  lateral wall
  posterior wall
Abnormal shadows

3. Gas shadows

Within alimentary tract:
  normal
  abnormal
Within peritoneal cavity
Other abnormal sites

4. Opacities

5. General view

1. The bones

Every bone should be studied, noting particularly the adjacent joint and disc spaces, the inner and outer layers of the cortex, and the trabecular pattern. The density of the bone and areas of lysis or sclerosis should be assessed.

Common variations that may cause confusion are:

(a) 'Lumbarization' of the first part of the sacrum;
(b) 'Sacralization' of the last lumbar vertebra;
(c) L.5 or S.1 spina bifida: Fig. 64;
(d) The epiphysis of a transverse process of a lumber vertebra;
(e) Calcification in costal cartilages which may be random and irregular and occurs even in young adults. On the plain abdominal film it may overlie visceral soft tissue shadows in the upper abdomen.

Inspection of the bones on the abdominal film is particularly important in patients who have been injured, as fractures, e.g. of a transverse process of a lumbar vertebra, may be discovered (Fig. 59). This fracture, unimportant in itself, should sugest the possibility of a renal or other intra-abdominal injury.

In other patients with abdominal pain unsuspected bony changes may be found which point to the diagnosis, e.g. a collapsed vertebral body due to malignant deposits may produce root pain, simulating an acute abdominal condition (Fig. 64).

2. Soft tissue shadows

Viscera

The outlines of the liver, spleen, kidneys and bladder should be sought. Any abnormality of size, position or margin must be noted, e.g. an adrenal tumour whilst not being visible itself on plain X-ray, may displace the kidney downwards; on the left an aortic aneurysm may displace the kidney laterally.

Figure 1: Normal liver, spleen and kidneys.

Figure 2: Riedel's lobe of liver.

Figure 3: Enlarged spleen.

Abdominal wall

The height and shape of the diaphragm on each side may reflect changes either in the underlying abdominal viscera or subphrenic spaces, or in the overlying lung (e.g. lobar collapse).

The 'flank stripe' is an important landmark in the lateral abdominal wall (Fig. 2). Its translucency represents the layer of extraperitoneal fat in the flank and is delineated laterally by the abdominal muscles and medially by the peritoneum and abdominal contents. The stripe may be obliterated by the oedema of an inflammatory mass involving the abdominal wall.

The lateral border of the psoas muscle provides a landmark on the posterior abdominal wall (Fig. 1) and may be similarly wholly or partly obliterated by adjacent inflammation or retroperitoneal haemorrhage.

Abnormal shadows

Many intra-abdominal diseases produce abnormal soft tissue shadows, e.g. abscesses and aneurysms. The position, size, shape and density of these shadows must be observed (Figs 21 and 23). Some soft tissue shadows may include areas of calcification (Fig. 84). Others which are fat-containing, e.g. lipomata or ovarian cysts (Fig. 55) may be less dense (i.e. darker) than surrounding soft tissue structures. Further examples of abnormal soft tissue shadows are illustrated in later chapters (Figs 15, 37, 40, 56, etc.).

3. Gas shadows

There are three relevant points to be noted.

(i) *Whether the gas is within the intestinal tract*

The small bowel and large bowel mucosal patterns are characteristic and often are well outlined by contained gas. The outline of gas in the stomach fundus is also characteristic, a point which assists in its differentiation from free gas in the peritoneal cavity (Fig. 5). There are variable amounts of gas in the different parts of the gut in the normal state, the small bowel in the adult usually containing little air. In the normal young child or in the bed-ridden aged patient apparently excessive amounts of small bowel gas are seen (Fig. 65). Admixture of air and semifluid or semiformed faeces produces a characteristic speckled appearance in the large bowel (Fig. 66). This appearance is only seen in the small bowel in exceptional circumstances, e.g. Fig. 75 (mucoviscidosis).

(ii) *Whether the gas is free in the peritoneal cavity*

If the gas is free note its site. Unless it is present in large amounts free gas will usually be detected only in the erect (vertical) or lateral decubitus film (Figs 5 and 6), and for a reliable result the patient should have been in this position for at least 5 min before the radiograph is taken. Occasionally in the supine film free gas will be seen outlining the lower border of the liver, or the outside as well as the inside of a loop of bowel (Fig. 7). Free gas in the lesser sac may be difficult to diagnose. In the erect film it may show up as a gas collection behind the stomach 2 to 5 cm below the diaphragm. If the patient is turned on the left side the gas may pass through the aditus to the lesser sac and be more readily seen in the lateral decubitus view.

(iii) *Whether the gas is in other abnormal sites*

The commonest abnormal site is in a subphrenic abscess (Fig. 38). Other examples are gas in the biliary tree (Figs 17 and 18), portal venous system, intestinal wall (Figs 29 and 79) or layers of the abdominal wall or pelvis. Gas may tract into the lower limb from an extraperitoneal perforation of the large bowel and present an appearance suggestive of gas gangrene (Fig. 30).

4. Opacities

Many different opacities may be seen on the plain abdominal X-ray. Their site, size, density and outline must be noted. The relevance of these factors, with examples, will be discussed in Chapter 6. Some opacities will prove to be variations of normal, e.g. costochondral calcification or phleboliths, or incidental to the problem of abdominal pain, e.g. a calcified fibroid.

5. General view

Having examined the films at a normal viewing distance step back to about five feet (1.5 m) from the viewing box to obtain a general view of the film. Paradoxically, gross changes may sometimes be missed unless this is done.

Normal bowel gas pattern in the adult
Fig. 1

X-RAY APPEARANCES
(Supine film)

Gas in the stomach (arrowed).
Gas in the hepatic flexure, splenic flexure, descending colon and sigmoid colon.
Minimal gas in the small intestine.
Calcified costal cartilages, best seen on the right.
Outline of the upper part of the right kidney and lower pole of the left kidney.
Left psoas margin seen better than right.

There is a slight degree of scoliosis, convex to the left. This appearance in a supine film is usually due to the patient lying with some lateral flexion. However, in the investigation of a patient with abdominal pain scoliosis may be produced by inflammatory lesions involving the posterior abdominal wall (e.g. perinephric abscess), by trauma (e.g. fractured transverse process of a vertebra, see Fig. 59) or by acute prolapse of an intervertebral disc, all of which produce spasm of the adjacent muscles.

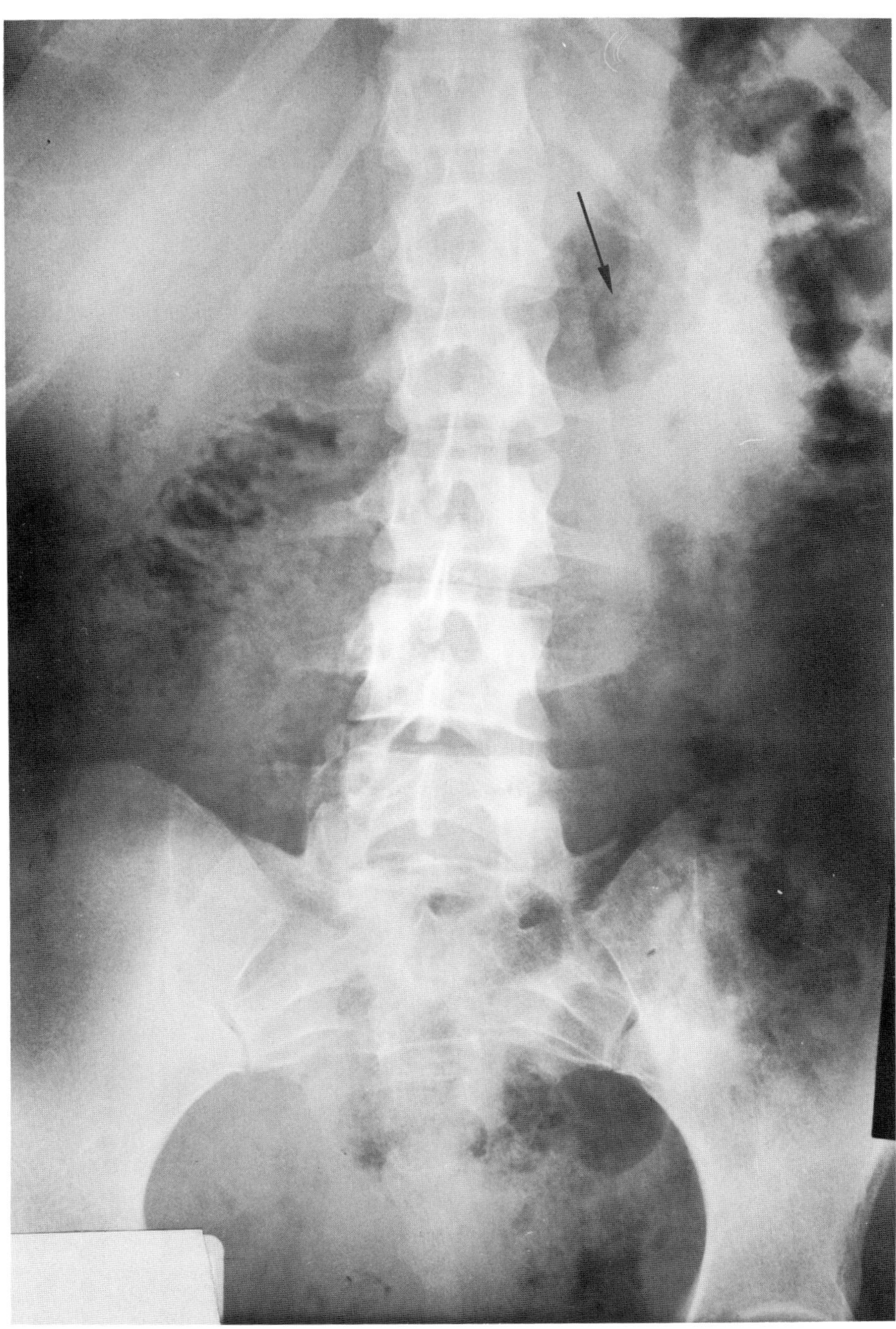

Fig. 1. Normal bowel gas pattern and normal kidneys.

Normal appearance—Riedel's lobe of the liver
Fig. 2

X-RAY APPEARANCE
(Supine film)

Tongue like projection (arrowed) of the right lobe of the liver (Riedel's lobe) displacing the hepatic flexure of the colon downwards and medially.
Normal right kidney shadow.
Clear right flank stripe.
Calcified costal cartilages.
Soft tissue shadow (arrowed) produced by the skin fold at the waist when the patient is supine.

This process of the liver is a variation of the normal shape, and has no clinical significance. It is commoner in women, and when present must be differentiated both radiologically and clinically from a hepatic, renal or colonic mass.

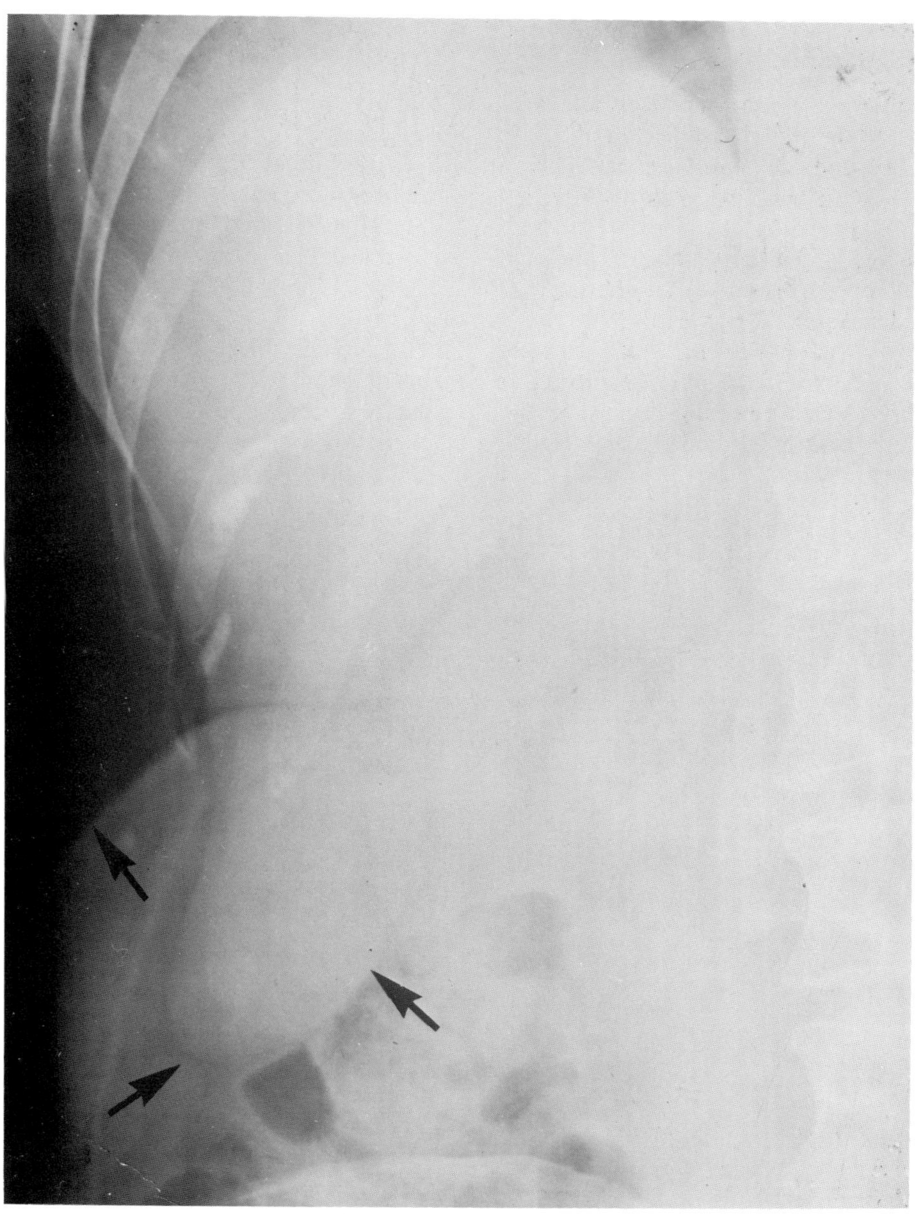

Fig. 2. Riedel's lobe of the liver.

Enlarged spleen
Fig. 3

X-RAY APPEARANCES (Supine film)

Enlarged spleen, the lower pole being at the level of the iliac crest.

The stomach is displaced medially and the splenic flexure of the colon downwards.

The granular appearance of the gastric contents is somewhat unusual but normal.

The notch on the anterior splenic border may be visible because of the fatty contrast provided by the greater omentum.

DIFFERENTIAL DIAGNOSIS OF X-RAY

Enlarged left kidney: excretory urography will differentiate.

CLINICAL DIFFERENTIAL DIAGNOSIS

Massive splenic enlargement may be caused by:

chronic myeloid leukaemia, myelofibrosis, thalassaemia, portal hypertension, malarial infestation, lipoid storage diseases and rarely splenic cysts.

Clinically the spleen is palpable centrally and towards the right iliac fossa: radiographically its axis frequently appears more vertical.

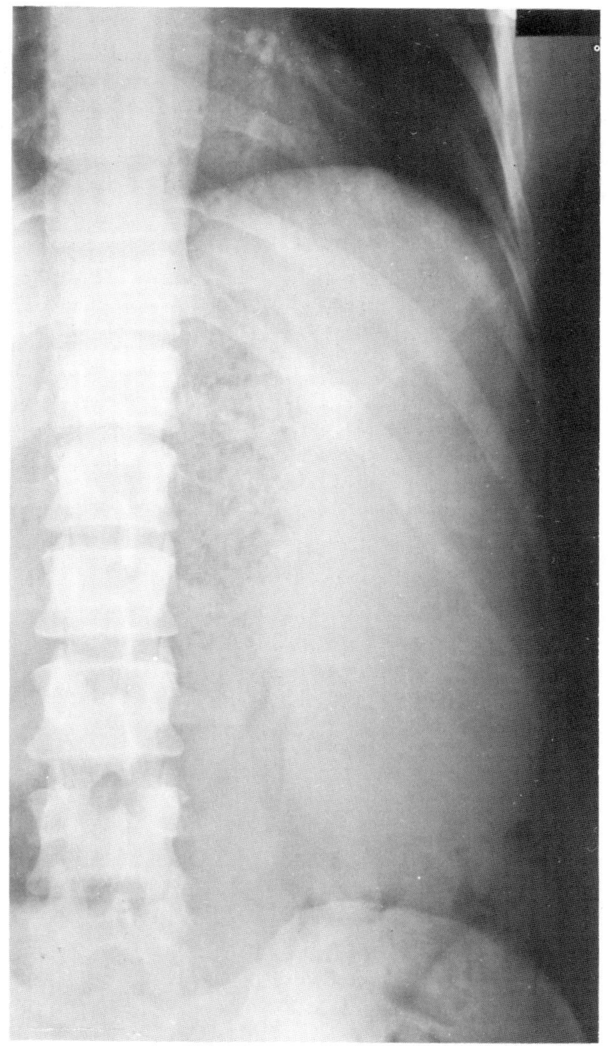

Fig. 3. Enlarged spleen.

Chapter 2
Alimentary System

In the majority of patients presenting with an acute abdominal emergency the causative lesion is to be found in the alimentary tract or one of its associated structures, such as the pancreas. The history and clinical examination are of the greatest importance, and on occasion laboratory tests may be helpful. The decision as to whether or not to operate, and with what degree of urgency, is sometimes difficult and it is often the plain abdominal and chest X-rays which provide the deciding information. As previously mentioned, the chest X-ray may not only suggest that the abdominal pain is referred from the chest, e.g. lobar pneumonia (Fig. 42) or spontaneous perforation of the oesophagus (Fig. 4), but may also provide other, unexpected information regarding the patient's general condition, e.g. an enlarged heart or pulmonary metastases. In a patient with a subphrenic abscess (Fig. 38), or even acute cholecystitis, coincident abnormality of the chest film may be noted, e.g. basal collapse or a sympathetic pleural effusion.

Gas and fluid are usually present in increased quantity in the dilated intestinal loops proximal to an obstruction, and fluid levels are a well known and valuable sign on plain X-ray. However, it may be some hours after the onset of obstruction before there are abnormal X-ray appearances. The presence of fluid levels does not invariably indicate obstruction for they may be found in patients who have gastroenteritis; who have recently taken a laxative such as magnesium sulphate which increases the fluid content of the intestine; or in a patient who has recently had an enema when fluid levels in the large bowel may persist for 2–4 hours. Such large bowel fluid levels only assume significance if they persist beyond this time.

In contrast, the absence of fluid levels does not always exclude the diagnosis of obstruction. In high jejunal obstruction the vomiting may start so early in the course of the disease, and be so profuse, that the intestine proximal to the obstruction is emptied and the plain X-ray may appear misleadingly normal (Fig. 24 legend). Similarly, a distended loop of bowel filled with fluid and without gas will not show a gas-fluid level: an acute volvulus of the small intestine around a band may show solely as a localized area of increased density.

A single loop of dilated bowel may be found adjacent to an inflamed viscus—the 'sentinel loop' (Fig. 22)—and on erect film this loop may show a fluid level. This represents an example of localized paralytic (adynamic) ileus, and is a valuable X-ray sign.

Generalized paralytic (adynamic) ileus may follow abdominal operation, peritoneal sepsis, retro-peritoneal haemorrhage or vertebral injury. Radiographically the appearance of numerous dilated loops of small and large bowel, with fluid levels, may be very similar to that of mechanical obstruction, but auscultation of the patient's abdomen will differentiate the two conditions. After a mesenteric vascular accident, e.g. superior mesenteric artery embolus, functional paralysis of intestinal loops soon ensues and the characteristic X-ray appearance is one of multiple dilated small bowel loops, with fluid levels (Fig. 20).

The patient complaining of acute abdominal pain in the postoperative period presents a difficult diagnostic problem. Air under the diaphragm introduced at laparotomy, or loops of small bowel with air-fluid levels due to paralytic (adynamic) ileus, will complicate the interpretation of the plain films. **In this and other circumstances the absence of clear radiographic signs should not deter the surgeon from laparotomy if indicated by the clinical features.** For example, the absence of free air under the diaphragm in a patient presenting clinically as a perforated peptic ulcer should not alter the diagnosis.

There is a number of medical diseases in which abdominal pain may uncommonly be a presenting symptom. Examples include migraine, herpes zoster, porphyria, epidemic myalgia, tabes dorsalis, and acute diabetes mellitus. An unexpectedly normal abdominal radiograph should alert the clinician to the possibility of one of these diagnoses.

Perforation of the oesophagus Figs 4a and b

X-RAY APPEARANCES

Fig. 4a

Gas in the tissue planes of the neck (arrowed).
Delineation of the parietal pleura by mediastinal gas (arrowed).

Fig. 4b

Gas in the tissue planes of the neck (arrowed) and mediastinum.
Pneumothorax on the right (lung margin arrowed).
Bilateral pleural effusion, with fluid level on the right.

Fluid levels are only seen with an effusion if there is an associated pneumothorax. Subdiaphragmatic gas may sometimes be seen.

DIFFERENTIAL DIAGNOSIS OF X-RAY

Spontaneous perforation of the oesophagus.
Endoscopic or surgical perforation of the oesophagus or trachea.
Chest trauma producing surgical emphysema.
Spontaneous pneumothorax.
Extra-pleural rupture of a bulla in status asthmaticus.
Subphrenic or lung abscess (a pneumothorax having been induced by attempts at diagnostic aspiration).

An X-ray examination using swallowed water soluble contrast medium may prove the diagnosis if this is in doubt and may demonstrate the site of the perforation.

PRESENTATION

History of an endoscopic examination especially when stricture dilatation has been performed; or following an attack of vomiting or coughing in the previous 24 h (Boerhaave's syndrome). Pain develops in the chest and back and radiates to the neck or to the abdomen. Shock ensues: surgical emphysema provides the clue to the diagnosis.

CLINICAL DIFFERENTIAL DIAGNOSIS

Myocardial infarction.
Perforated peptic ulcer.
Acute pancreatitis.
Leak or dissection of an aortic aneurysm.
Pulmonary embolus.
Pneumonia.
Pericarditis.
Spontaneous pneumothorax.
Mallory–Weiss syndrome.

(a)

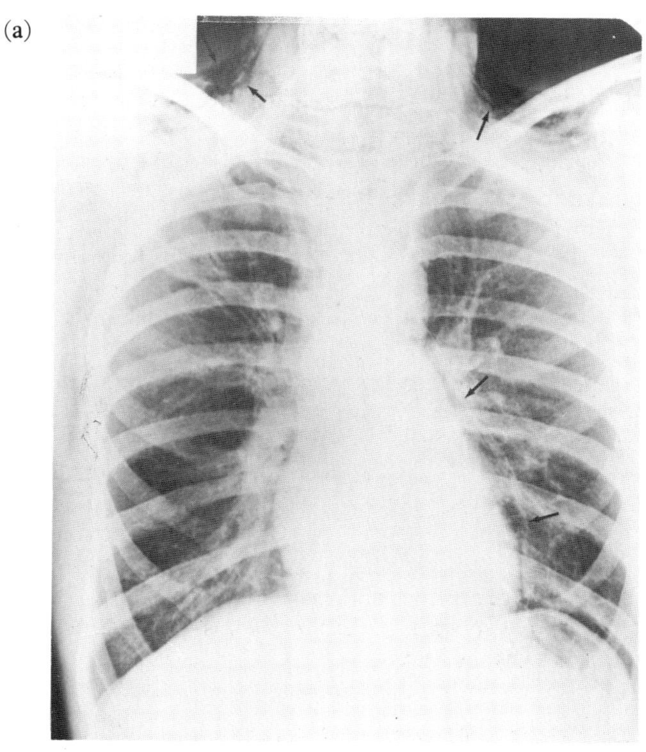

(b)

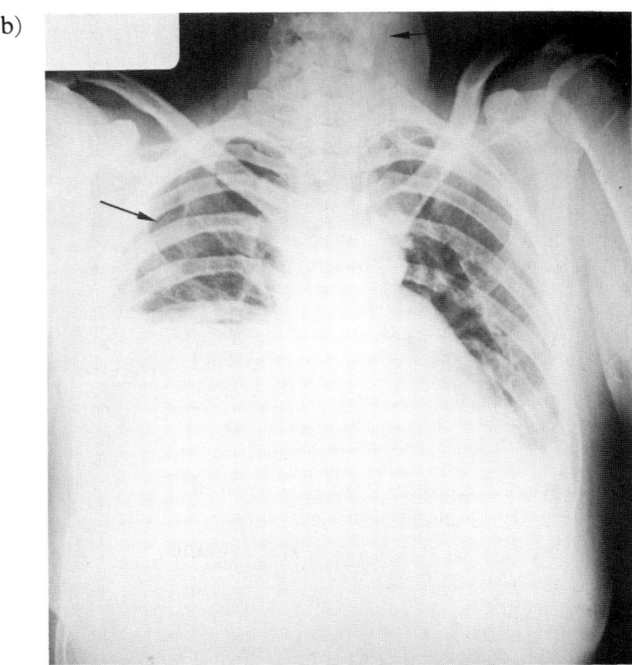

Fig. 4. Perforation of oesophagus.

Perforated peptic ulcer
Fig. 5

X-RAY APPEARANCES
(Erect film)

Free gas between the liver and the right side of the diaphragm.

Difficulty in deciding whether gas is free or in the stomach fundus will be resolved by inspecing a lateral decubitus (left uppermost film, Fig. 6). Free gas is not visible on X-ray in about a third of patients with a perforated peptic ulcer. In these a water soluble contrast meal may demonstrate the perforation.

DIFFERENTIAL DIAGNOSIS OF X-RAY

Perforation of any part of the gut (most commonly a peptic ulcer or of a colonic diverticulum).
Laparotomy within the previous fourteen days.
Spontaneous rupure of a gas cyst of the intestine (Fig. 25).
Subphrenic abscess (Fig. 38).
Tubal insufflation within the previous 24 h.
Introduction of air at peritoneal dialysis, laparoscopy, peritoneal lavage or by a penetrating woud.
Interposition of a distended bowel loop between the diaphragm and the liver (Chilaiditi's syndrome, Fig. 8).

PRESENTATION

Sudden onset of acute upper abdominal pain in a patient who may, **or may not,** have had a history of dyspepsia.
Signs of peritonitis, including 'board-like' rigidity, and sometimes loss of liver dullness.

Atypical presentation is not uncommon, e.g. gradual onset of pain; absence of 'board-like' rigidity; right iliac fossa pain and tenderness due to spillage into the right paracolic gutter. Symptoms and signs may be masked in the aged and in those receiving steroid therapy.

Perforation of the appendix seldom produces free intraperitoneal gas.

CLINICAL DIFFERENTIAL DIAGNOSIS

Acute exacerbation of a peptic ulcer.
Acute gastritis.
Acute pancreatitis.
Small bowel obstruction, particularly with infarction.
Mesenteric vascular accident.
Acute appendicitis and other causes of peritonitis.
Leak or dissection of an aortic aneurysm.
Myocardial infarction.
Acute cholecystitis.
Bile duct or ureteric colic.
Perforation of the oesophagus.

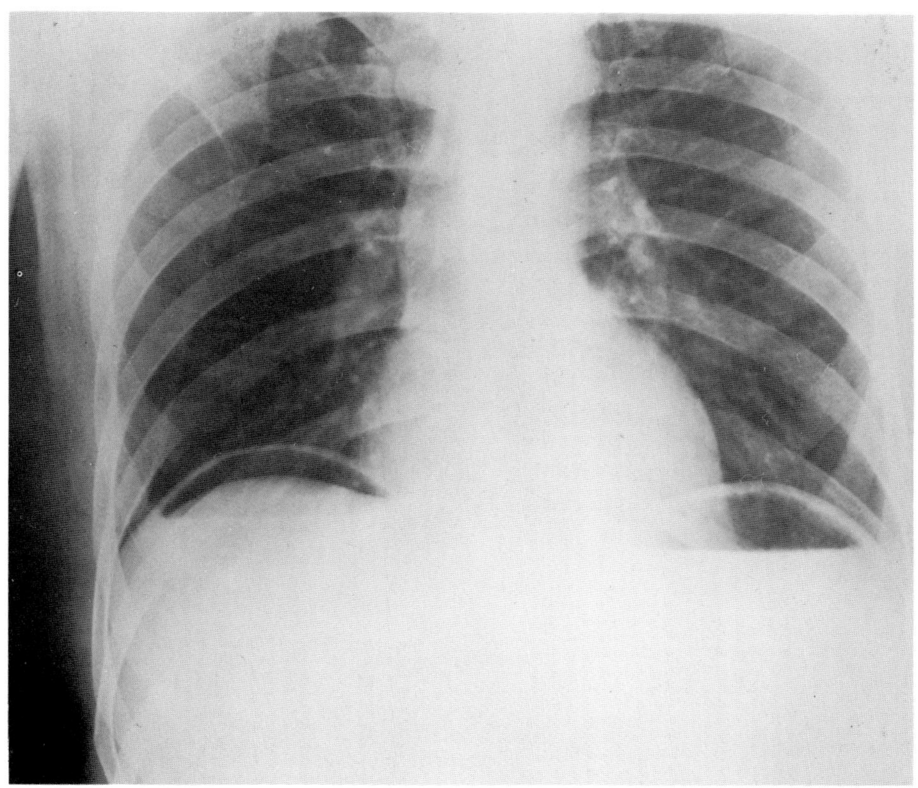

Fig. 5. Perforated peptic ulcer (erect).

Perforated peptic ulcer
Fig. 6

X-RAY APPEARANCES
(Left lateral erect film)

Free gas under the left side of the diaphragm.

In this patient the splenic shadow is visible (arrowed) below the gas.

Overlying the splenic shadow small amounts of gas are seen in the splenic flexure of the colon and the gastric fundus.

Generalized 'ground glass' appearance suggesting excessive free peritoneal fluid (Fig. 40).

The irregular linear shadows on the inferior aspect of the film are produced by folds of clothing or bedding.

Such artefacts often obscure detail in the lower part of a lateral erect film, but this area can be seen in the film with the other side uppermost. The free gas could not be in the stomach fundus unless the patient had previously had a splenectomy. A lateral erect film should be taken only after the patient has been in this position for several minutes to allow the air to ascend to the highest point in the abdomen.

PRESENTATION AND DIFFERENTIAL DIAGNOSIS

See Fig. 5 legend.

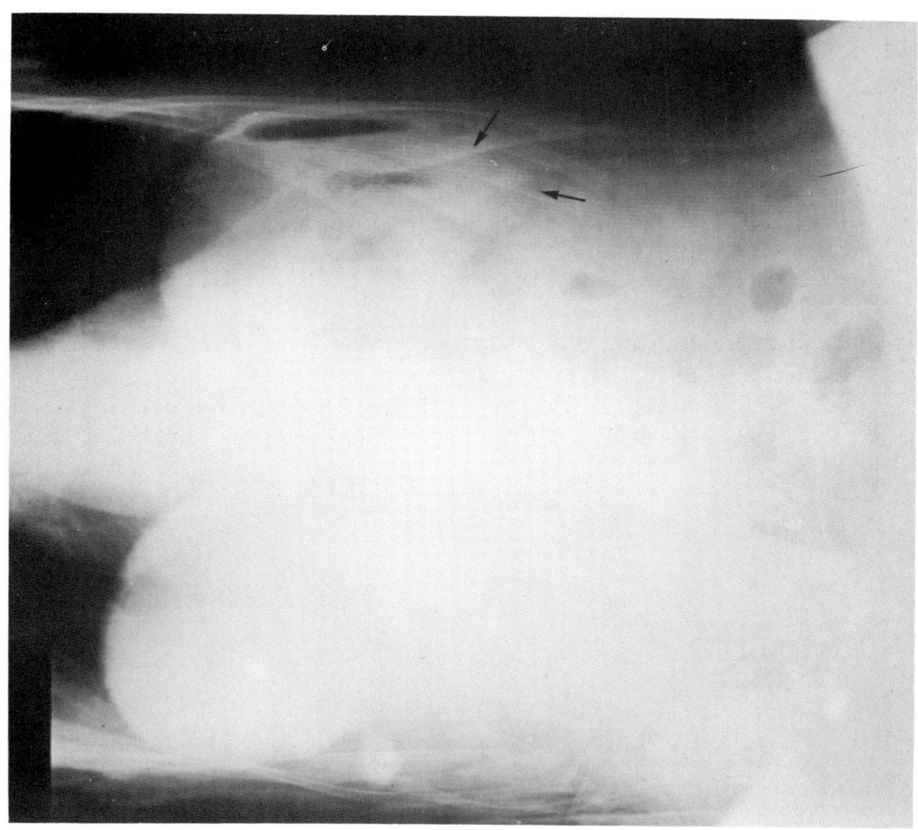

Fig. 6. Perforated peptic ulcer.

Perforated peptic ulcer
Fig. 7

X-RAY APPEARANCES

(Erect film)

Gross pneumoperitoneum.

Intraperitoneal air-fluid level, arrowed (1).

Free gas separating gas-filled loops of bowel, arrowed (2). ('The bas relief sign').

Distended loops of bowel with fluid levels, arrowed (3).

Irregular gas outlines in the subhepatic spaces, arrowed (4).

Gas lateral to the liver.

DIFFERENTIAL DIAGNOSIS OF X-RAY

Perforation of any part of the gut, especially of the stomach after a large meal, or when diagnosis has been delayed.

PRESENTATION

See Fig. 5 legend.

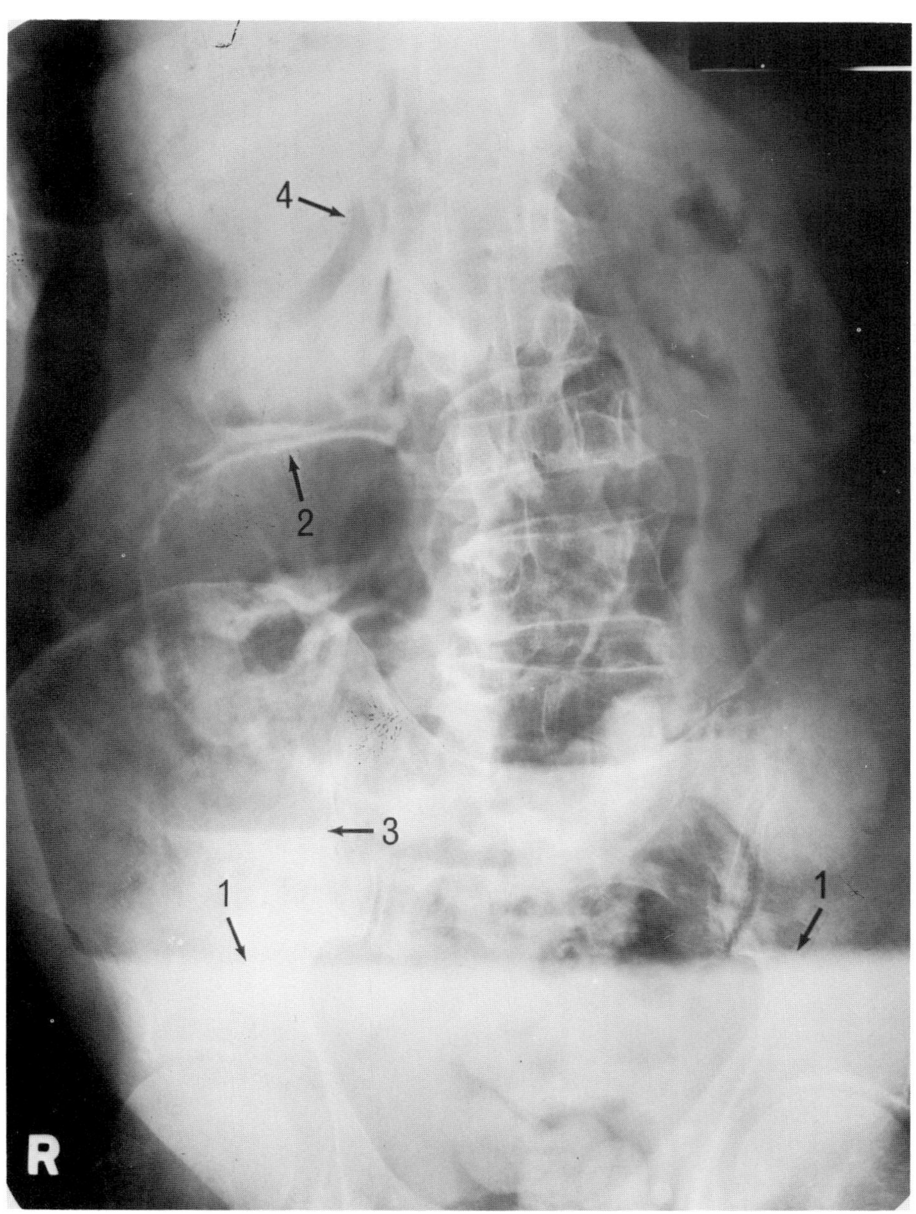

Fig. 7. Perforated peptic ulcer.

Chilaiditi's syndrome and perforated peptic ulcer Fig. 8

X-RAY APPEARANCES

Elevation of part of the right hemidiaphragm.
Loop of colon interposed between the liver and the diaphragm.
Free intraperitoneal gas under the right hemidiaphragm.
Soft tissue shadow of the liver below the interposed colon.

Chilaiditi's syndrome (or subphrenic interposition) refers to the presence of a colonic loop or less frequently a small intestinal loop between the liver and the diaphragm. The condition is sometimes associated with abnormalities of the hepatic ligaments, but often is of no clinical importance.

DIFFERENTIAL DIAGNOSIS OF X-RAY

Diaphragmatic hernia.
Ruptured diaphragm.
Free intraperitoneal gas may be due to a number of causes—see legend to Fig. 5.

CLINICAL PRESENTATION

In adults usually asymptomatic.
In children: abdominal pain and distension, typically at the end of the day, and relieved by lying down.
Aerophagy.
Less frequent symptoms include anorexia, constipation and passage of excessive amounts of flatus.

For presentation of perforated peptic ulcer, see legend to Fig. 5.

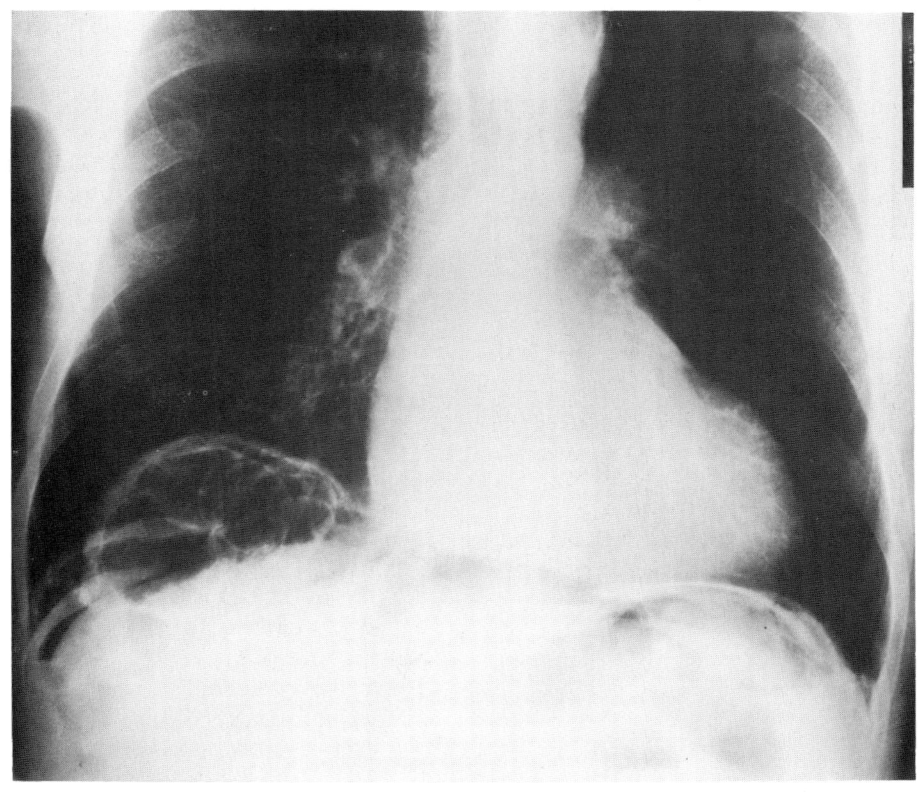

Fig. 8. Chilaiditi's syndrome and perforated peptic ulcer.

Acute gastric dilatation
Fig. 9a and b

X-RAY APPEARANCES
(Erect and supine film)

Stomach grossly distended with air and fluid, occupying the whole of the upper abdomen.
Gastric fluid level on the erect film.
Distended jejunal loop, again with fluid levels, on the erect film.

In this patient the jejunal dilatation is due to coincident paralytic ileus.

DIFFERENTIAL DIAGNOSIS OF X-RAY

Volvulus of the stomach.
Pneumoperitoneum.
Pyloric stenosis.

PRESENTATION

Epigastric pain and distension.
Severe nausea.
Pallor, sweating, tachycardia.
Air swallowing and belching. This may be initiated by nausea produced by some other condition, for example acute appendicitis or post-operative paralytic ileus.

Acute gastric distension commonly occurs post-operatively and after abdominal trauma and is due to air swallowing.

CLINICAL DIFFERENTIAL DIAGNOSIS

Volvulus of the stomach or colon.
Perforation of a viscus.
Pyloric stenosis.
Intestinal obstruction.
Gram-negative septicaemia.

(a)

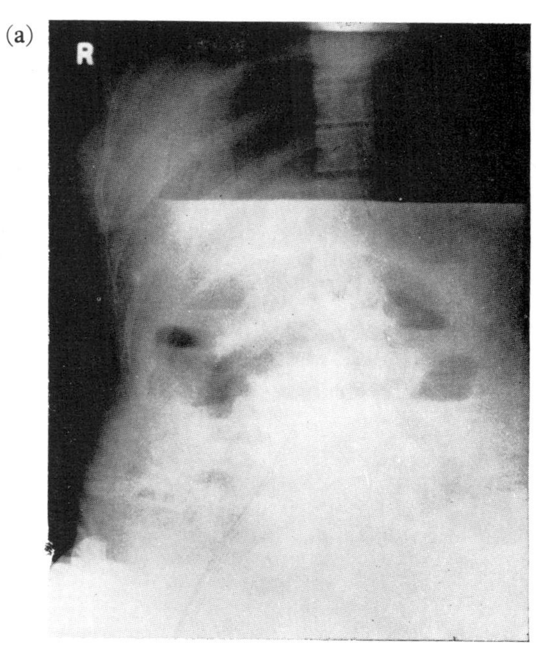

(b)

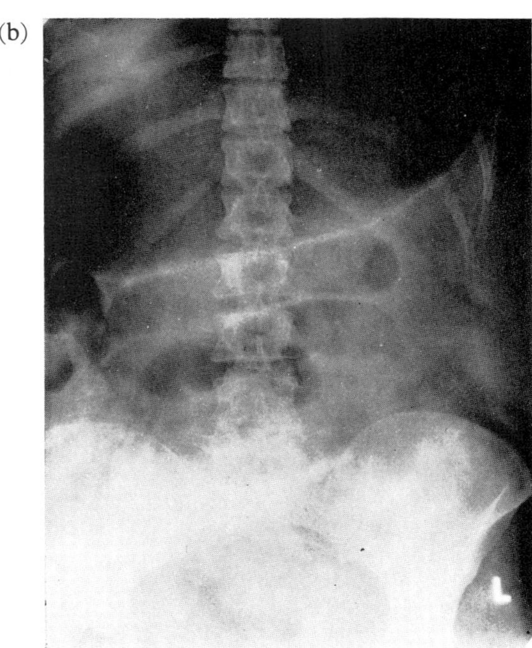

Fig. 9. Acute gastric dilatation: (a) erect and (b) supine.

Gastric foreign body
Fig. 10

X-RAY APPEARANCES
(Supine film)

Coin in the gastric antrum.
The greater curvature of the filled stomach is 'outlined' by the gas in the transverse colon.

DIFFERENTIAL DIAGNOSIS OF X-RAY

Concerns only the site of the foreign body.

PRESENTATION

History of swallowing foreign body.
Occasional vomiting, without pain.

The great majority of swallowed foreign bodies pass through the gut spontaneously without causing symptoms.

This is also the case in children, but to reduce both parental anxiety and the number of check radiographs endoscopic removal of the foreign body is often undertaken.

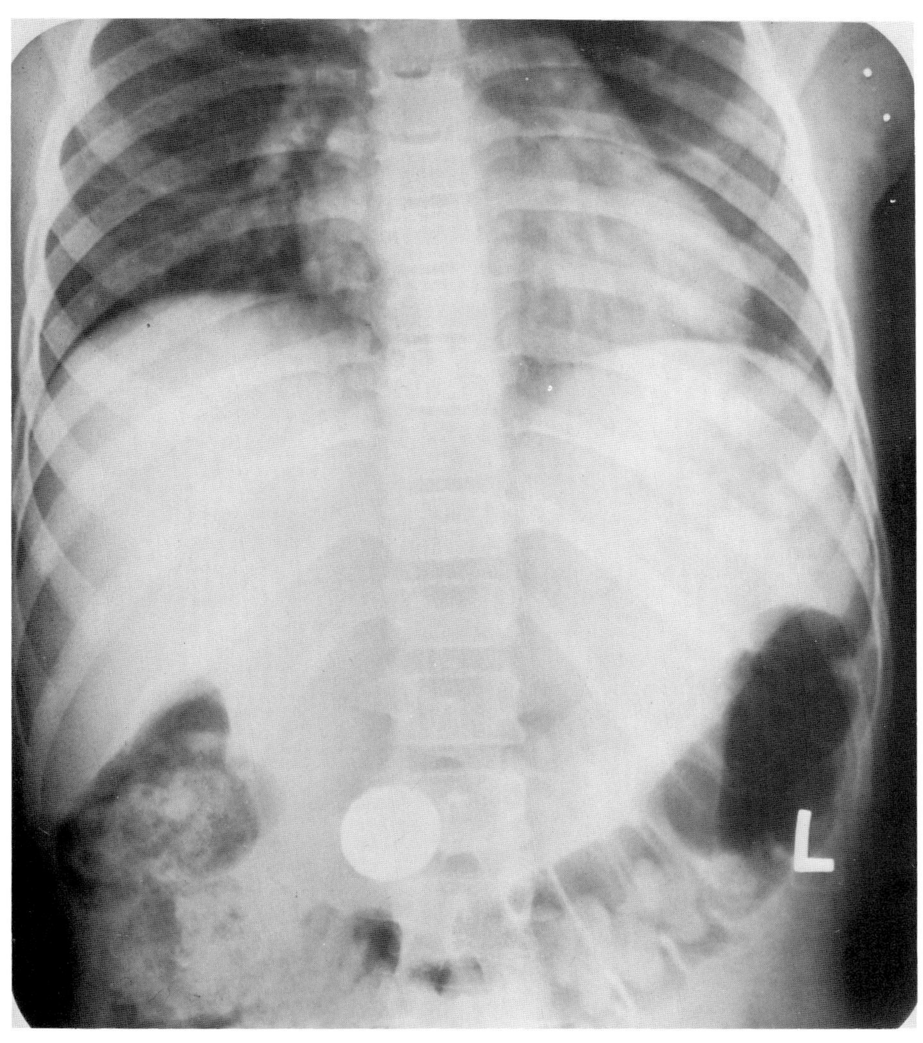

Fig. 10. Gastric foreign body.

Duodenal diverticulum
Fig. 11

X-RAY APPEARANCES
(**Supine film**)

Circular translucency to the left of L2–3 intervertebral space, arrowed.

The quantity of intragastric air is within normal limits.

DIFFERENTIAL DIAGNOSIS OF X-RAY

End-on view of a distended loop of small intestine. If so further distended loops would be expected.

The diagnosis was confirmed by barium meal. Duodenal diverticula occur most commonly in the second part of the duodenum.

PRESENTATION

As an incidental X-ray finding, as these diverticula are usually symptomless.

Diverticulitis or perforation is rare.

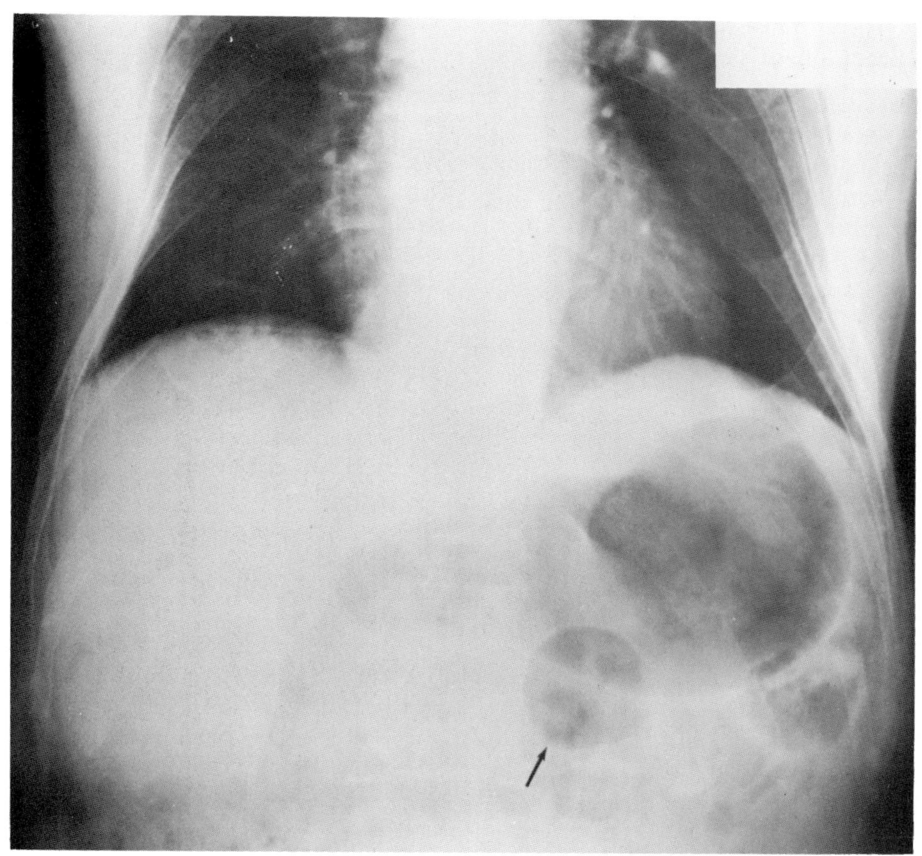

Fig. 11. Duodenal diverticulum.

Hiatus hernia
Fig. 12

X-RAY APPEARANCES
(Erect film of chest)

Gas filled fundus of the stomach with a fluid level, overlying the cardiac shadow and extending into the right hemithorax.
Calcification of costal cartilages—on the right more clearly shown through the fundal gas shadow.

Barium contrast studies later showed this to be a mixed rolling and sliding hiatus hernia.

DIFFERENTIAL DIAGNOSIS OF X-RAY

Mediastinal abscess.
Loculated empyema.
Achalasia of the cardia (with gross oesophageal dilatation).
Basal segmental collapse, if the presence of the hemispherical gas filled fundus is not appreciated.

PRESENTATION

Retrosternal discomfort or pain, especially after meals.
Dysphagia.
Weight loss.
Indigestion.
Recurrent chest infections due to aspiration.
Rarely, if there is a volvulus of the stomach, the presentation may be acute with severe central upper abdominal and chest pain.
Retching, with shock.
If surgery is delayed the stomach in the hiatus hernia may become gangrenous.

CLINICAL DIFFERENTIAL DIAGNOSIS

Myocardial ischaemia.
Oesophagitis or oesophageal spasm.
Gall bladder disease.
Oesophageal perforation.
Peptic ulcer.
Carcinoma of the stomach or pancreas.
Chronic pancreatitis.

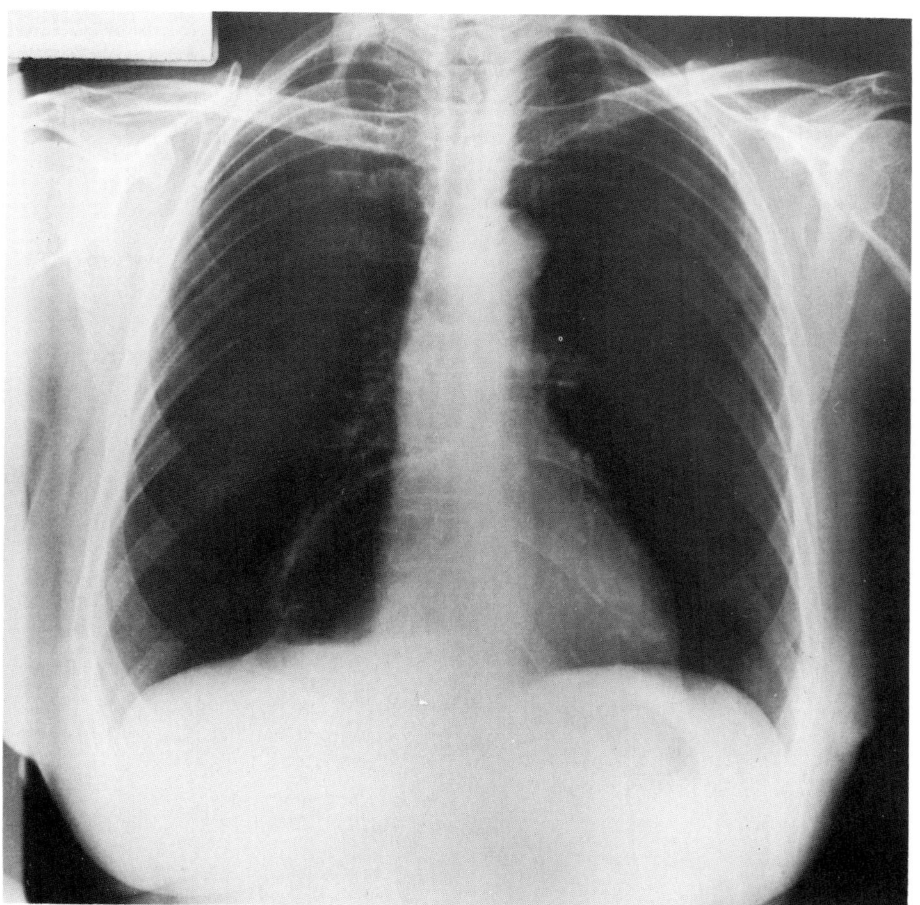

Fig. 12. Hiatus hernia.

Acute pancreatitis
Fig. 13

X-RAY APPEARANCES
(Lateral decubitus film, rightside uppermost)

C-shaped loop of moderately distended duodenum. The localized ileus results from contact with the inflamed head of pancreas.
Small fluid levels in the right iliac fossa representing early generalized paralytic ileus.
Absence of both psoas shadows due to retroperitoneal oedema.

The duodenal loop may on occasion show the 'reversed-3' or 'Epsilon' sign due to oedema of the head of the pancreas. The hepatic flexure of the colon may also show localized dilatation. Coincident sentinel loops of duodenum and transverse colon are virtually diagnostic of acute pancreatitis. There may sometimes be a small left pleural effusion.

As acute pancreatitis is frequently associated with disease of the biliary tract, gallstones may be seen either in the gallbladder or common duct on X-ray or ultrasound scan. Pancreatic calcification from previous episodes of pancreatitis may be evident (see Fig. 14).

A barium or gastrografin meal will demonstrate any duodenal abnormality.

DIFFERENTIAL DIAGNOSIS OF X-RAY

Acute cholecystitis.
Paralytic ileus associated with peritonitis.
Extrinsic obstruction of the third or fourth part of the duodenum due to haemorrhage or neoplasm.
Traumatic intramural haematoma or distal rupture of the duodenum.

PRESENTATION

Acute severe epigastric pain, often of sudden onset, radiating through to the back and sometimes to the chest.
Relief of pain may be obtained by bending forwards (unlike a perforated peptic ulcer).
Vomiting is profuse at first and followed by retching.
Past symptoms may indicate biliary tract disease.

Examination may suggest a perforated viscus but abdominal rigidity is often less marked and circulatory collapse is more profound. Bradycardia is often a feature. There may be tenderness in the left loin.

CLINICAL DIFFERENTIAL DIAGNOSIS

Perforation of a viscus.
Myocardial infarction.
Rupture of an abdominal aortic aneurysm.
Dissecting aneurysm.
High small bowel obstruction.
Acute cholecystitis or gallstone colic.
Mesenteric vascular accident.
Acute exacerbation of a peptic ulcer.
Splenic infarct.
Acute appendicitis.

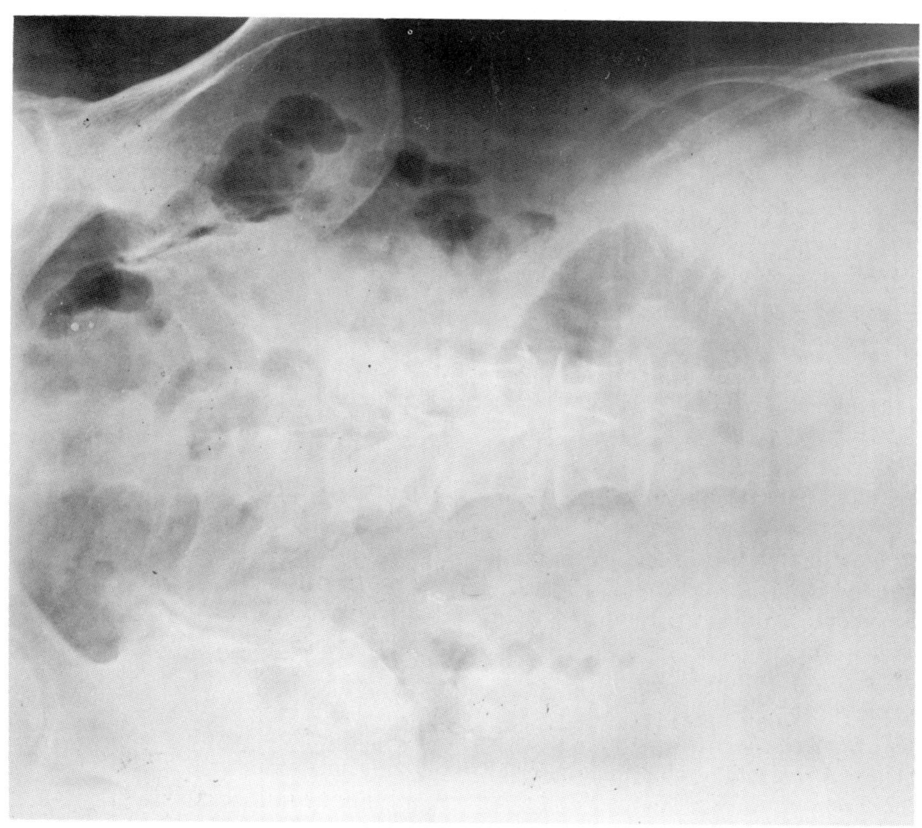

Fig. 13. Acute pancreatitis.

Chronic pancreatitis with calcification
Fig. 14

X-RAY APPEARANCES
(Film of epigastrium)

Patchy calcification concentrated in the head of the pancreas to the right of the 1st and 2nd lumbar vertebrae and extending into the body and tail.
The distribution of the calcification on the left suggests the presence of a cyst of the body of the pancreas, arrowed.
Gas-filled and somewhat dilated transverse colon.

Pancreatic calcification is present in only a minority of patients with chronic pancreatitis but when present it suggests a severe degree of destruction of pancreatic tissue. When calcification is seen on X-ray in a patient with acute upper abdominal pain it suggests the diagnosis of acute-on-chronic pancreatitis. Cyst formation in the pancreas indicates long-standing degenerative and obstructive changes; these patients may be diabetic or suffer from mal-absorption. In view of the association of pancreatic and biliary disease the film should be inspected for gallstones, and cholecystography or ultrasonography should be performed later. In parts of East Africa and India pancreatic calcification is common and is thought to be associated with malnutrition.

DIFFERENTIAL DIAGNOSIS OF X-RAY

Calcified lymph nodes.
Calcification in an aortic aneurysm.
Nephrocalcinosis.
Multiple renal calculi.
Adrenal calcification.

PRESENTATION

Recurrent symptoms suggesting mild acute pancreatitis (see legend to Fig. 13).
Back pain.
Diabetes mellitus.
Malabsorption syndrome.
Alcoholism and biliary tract disease are commonly associated.

CLINICAL DIFFERENTIAL DIAGNOSIS

Back pain due to spondylosis or metastatic deposits.
Carcinoma of the pancreas.
Abdominal aortic aneurysm.
Gallstone colic.
Mesenteric angina.
Cardiac angina.

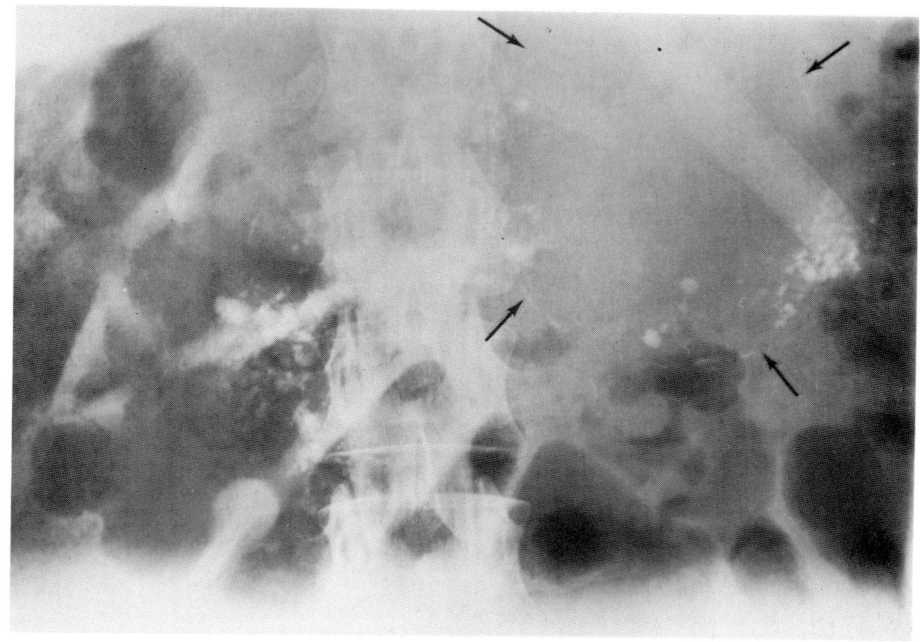

Fig. 14. Chronic pancreatitis with calcification.

Acute (emphysematous) cholecystitis—Gall bladder mass Fig. 15

X-RAY APPEARANCES (Supine)

Rim of gas outlining a soft tissue mass in the right upper quadrant (arrowed).
Gas in the biliary tree.

This uncommon appearance is due to infection of the gall bladder with a gas producing organism and occurs more frequently in diabetes. More commonly a soft tissue mass is seen with an associated sentinel loop of adjacent bowel.

DIFFERENTIAL DIAGNOSIS OF X-RAY

For gas in the biliary tract, see legend to Fig. 17.

PRESENTATION

Initially with the usual symptoms
of acute cholecystitis: right upper
abdominal or subcostal pain, radiating to the back, right shoulder or chest,
nausea or vomiting,
fever,
right upper quadrant tenderness and guarding, sometimes with an associated ill-defined mass.
If the wall of the gallbladder becomes gangrenous, as in this case:
rapid and progressive deterioration with shock, the development of generalized peritonitis with ileus,
jaundice.
See legend to Figs 17 and 18.

CLINICAL DIFFERENTIAL DIAGNOSIS

Perforation of a peptic ulcer with initial localization.
Inflammatory masses or abscesses originating from kidney, colon or appendix.
Liver abscess.
Acute pancreatitis.
Acute cholangitis.

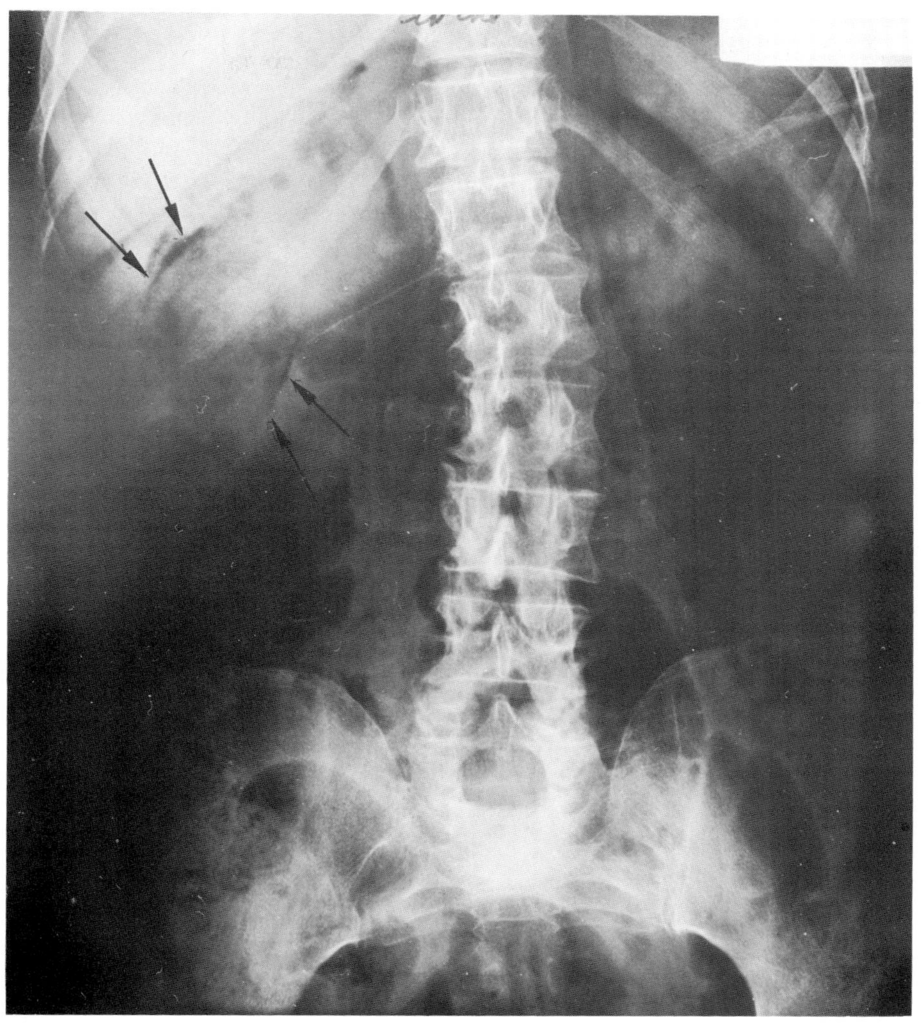

Fig. 15. Acute emphysematous cholecystitis—gall bladder mass.

Cholecystitis with gallstones Fig. 16

X-RAY APPEARANCES

Multiple gallstones in the fundus of a thick-walled gall bladder
Two gallstones, probably in Hartmann's pouch, arrowed.
Calcified mesenteric lymph gland at L.3 level.

The normal gall bladder rarely shows up on the plain X-ray, but if enlarged, e.g. a mucocele, it may indent the colonic gas shadow. Also, in chronic cholecystitis there is sometimes enough subserosal deposition of fat to provide a soft tissue outline of the gall bladder.

Only 10–15 per cent of all gallstones are visible on plain X-ray. They are usually 5–15 mm in diameter and are less dense than renal calculi. They may occasionally have a translucent centre. Ultrasonography usually provides the diagnosis without the need for contrast studies.

DIFFERENTIAL DIAGNOSIS OF X-RAY

Renal calculi. The lateral opacities are crossed by the renal outline; the medial opacities are within the renal shadow but their similar size, shape and density makes the diagnosis of renal calculi unlikely.
Ureteric calculus. The opacity at L.3 level lies in the line of the ureter. Its irregular outline and patchy calcification are typical of a calcified mesenteric gland. A lateral plain film will establish whether the opacity is on the posterior abdominal wall, and an excretory urogram will decide its relation to the ureter.

PRESENTATION AND CLINICAL DIFFERENTIAL DIAGNOSIS

See Fig. 15 legend.

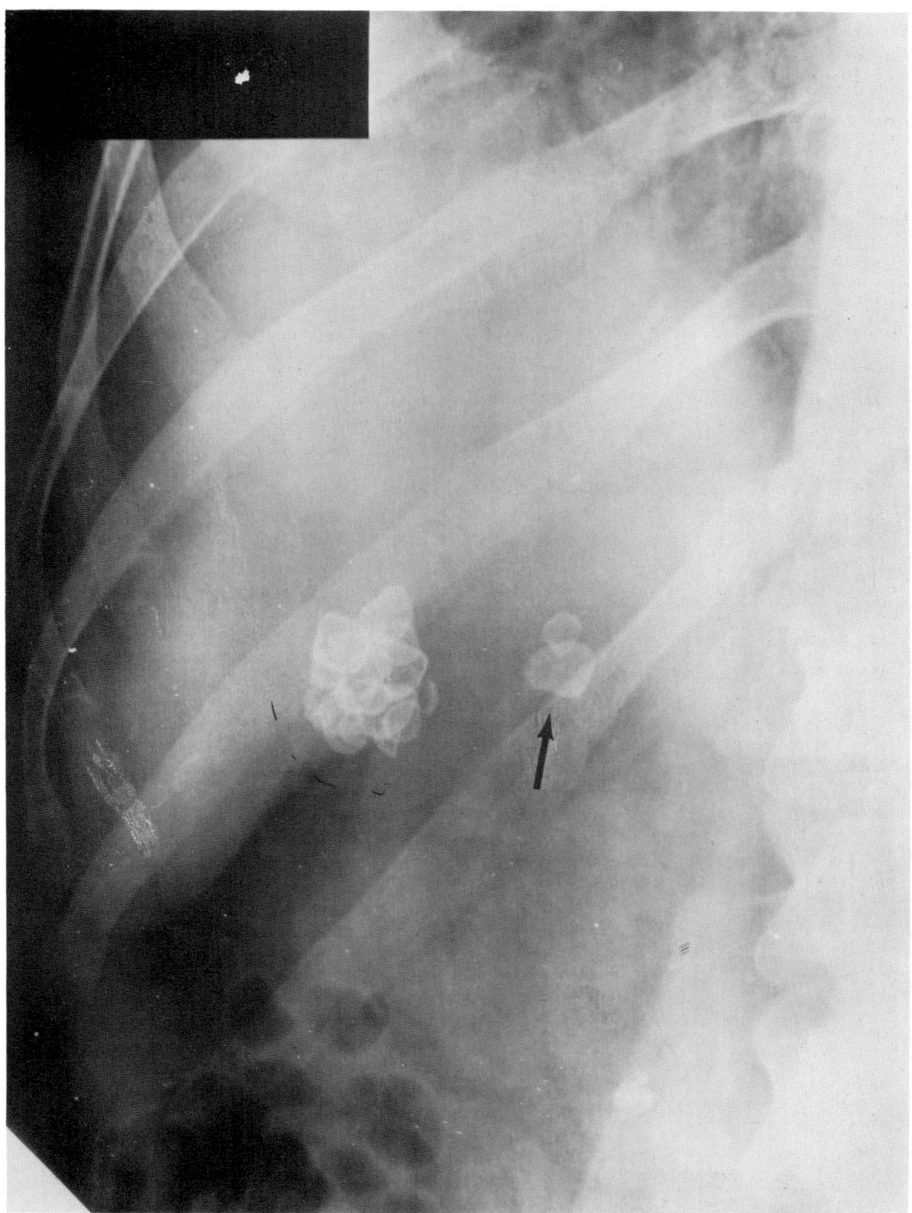

Fig. 16. Cholecystitis with gallstones.

Gas in the biliary system
Figs 17 and 18

X-RAY APPEARANCES

Fig. 17

Gas in the biliary tree, arrowed.
Gall bladder containing gas and a gallstone, arrowed.
Normal distribution of bowel gas.

Fig. 18: gallstone ileus

Gas in the biliary tree but not in the gall bladder, arrowed.
Distended loops of small intestine with fluid levels (see Fig. 80b).
Osteoarthritis of the right hip.
There is a suggestion of a large radio-opaque calculus opposite the right ischial spine. A localized view may show a calculus more clearly.

DIFFERENTIAL DIAGNOSIS OF X-RAY

Spontaneous fistula due to gallstone ulceration between the gall bladder

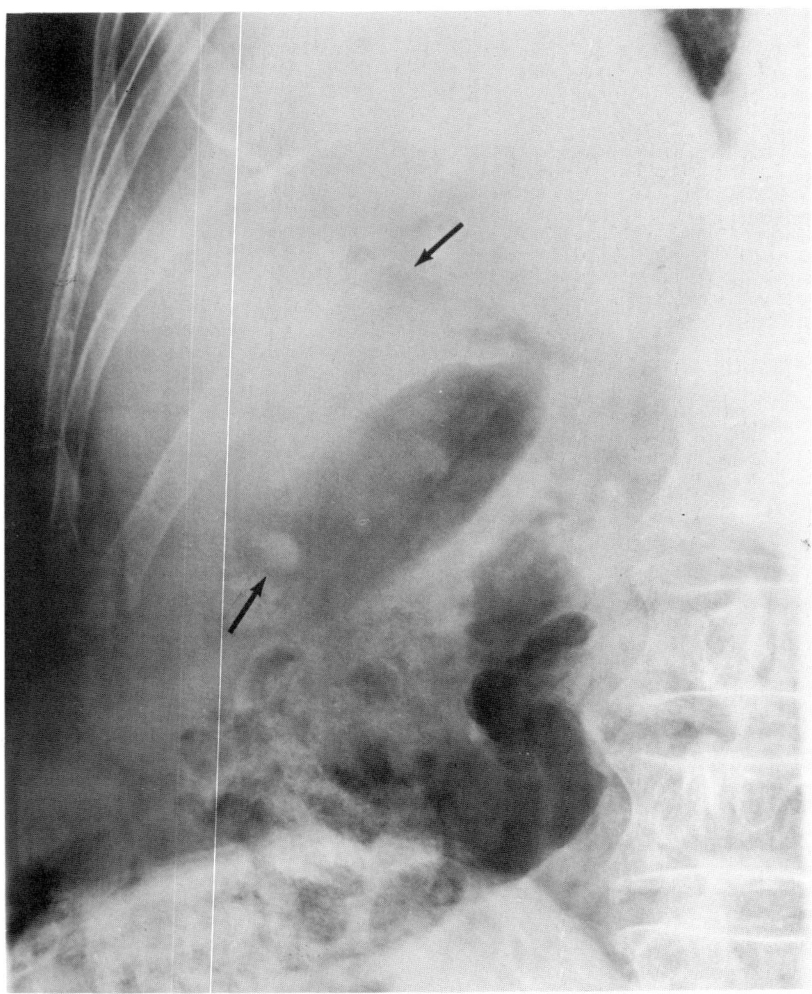

Fig. 17. Gas in the biliary system.

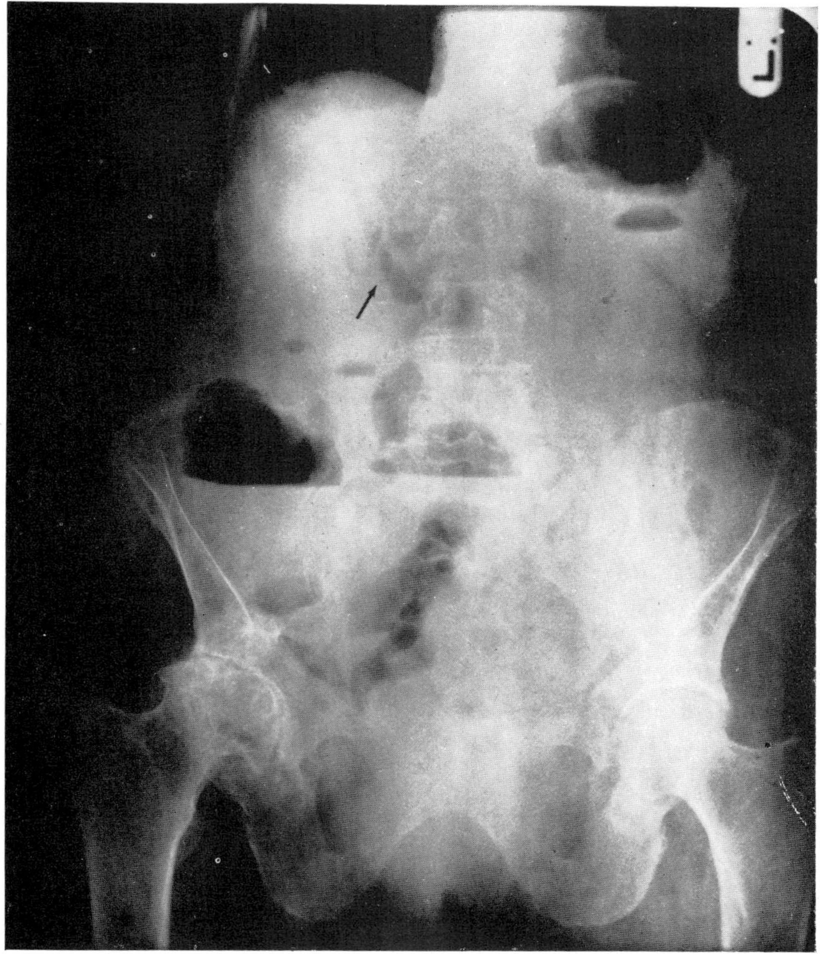

Fig. 18. Gas in the biliary system with gallstone ileus.

and the intestine, usually the duodenum.

Previous anastomosis between the gall bladder and the intestine, e.g. choledochoduodenostomy or cholecystjejunostomy.

Cholecystitis with gas-forming organisms.

Portal thrombophlebitis secondary to infection with gas-forming organisms.

PRESENTATION

This depends on the aetiology.

Figure 18 represents a patient with ileal obstruction due to an impacted gallstone.

If an anastomosis between the biliary tract and the gut is of sufficient size to allow free reflux and drainage of intestinal contents the presence of air in the biliary system is symptomless. If stenosis occurs cholangitis results and the patient will present with intermittent fever, rigors and jaundice.

The patient with gas-producing organisms infecting the gall bladder is usually a diabetic, is seriously ill, and has signs suggestive of acute cholecystitis.

Sickle cell crisis
Fig. 19

X-RAY APPEARANCES

(Supine film)
Increase in large and small bowel gas.
Multiple gallstones.
Decreased density of lumbar vertebrae.
Riedel's lobe displacing the ascending colon medially.
Soft tissue shadow of the penis overlying the pubic symphysis.

DIFFERENTIAL DIAGNOSIS OF X-RAY

Acute cholecystitis with secondary ileus.
Large bowel obstruction.
Intestinal pseudo obstruction.
Other causes of decreased bone density, e.g. thalassaemia, carcinomatosis, hyperparathyroidism, multiple myeloma, osteomalacia, osteoporosis (many causes).

PRESENTATION

This patient was a 22-year-old male Nigerian student with homozygous sickle cell anaemia.
Abdominal, back and chest pain.
Diarrhoea and vomiting.
Jaundice.
Anaemia.

Haemolysis in this condition causes the anaemia and jaundice and the hyperbilirubinaemia contributes to the formation of gallstones. Any patient of African origin with an acute abdomen should have a sickling test: when positive the result will be of importance if a general anaesthetic is required even if sickling is not directly the cause of the abdominal pain.

CLINICAL DIFFERENTIAL DIAGNOSIS

See legend to Fig. 15.

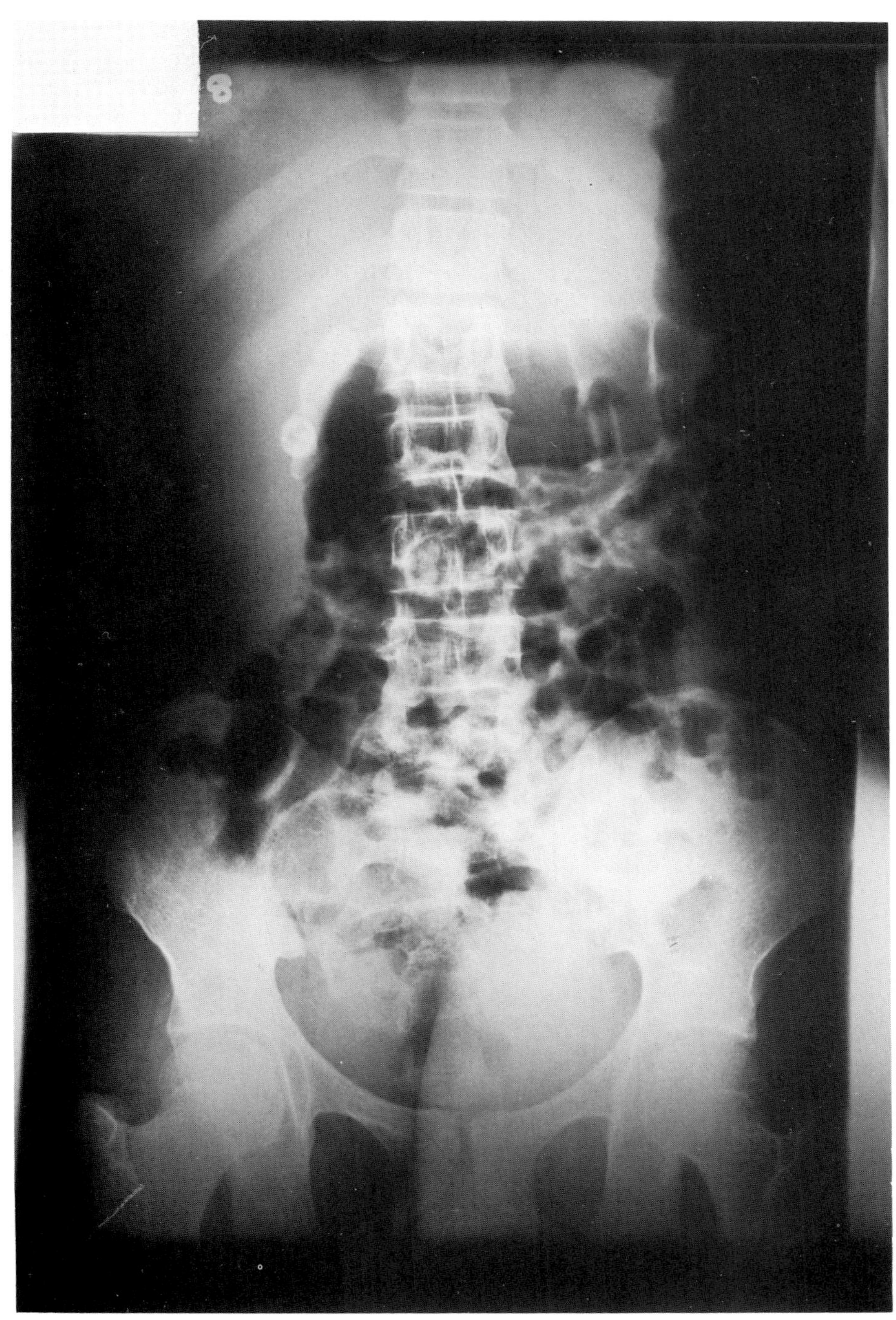

Fig. 19. Sickle cell crisis.

Paralytic (adynamic) ileus
Fig. 20

X-RAY APPEARANCES
(Supine film)

Generalized gaseous distension of both small and large bowel.
Loops of small bowel with mucosal folds continuous across their diameter, arrowed (1).
Distended transverse colon with haustra; the mucosal folds only partially cross the bowel diameter, arrowed (2).
Distended caecum, arrowed (3).
Sigmoid colon, arrowed (4); the absence of haustra in this segment of the colon may cause it to be confused with distended ileum.

DIFFERENTIAL DIAGNOSIS OF X-RAY

Mechanical obstruction of the colon or distal small bowel. Peritonitis causing paralytic ileus, in which case there may be no fluid between the loops of bowel.

If a patient with intestinal obstruction has been treated by the administration of an enema, fluid and air will be introduced distal to the obstructing lesion and may give an X-ray appearance similar to that of paralytic ileus.

Refer to Figs 21, 23, 24 and 27 for other differentiating features.

PRESENTATION

Abdominal distension.
Profuse vomiting.
Constipation.
Absence of colicky pain.
Diminished or absent bowel sounds.

The majority of cases are postoperative or associated with peritonitis.

CLINICAL DIFFERENTIAL DIAGNOSIS

Mechanical obstruction of small or large bowel.
Intestinal pseudo-obstruction (Fig. 28).
Metabolic disorders, e.g. uraemia, hypokalaemia.
Retroperitoneal haemorrhage, e.g. from fractured spine.

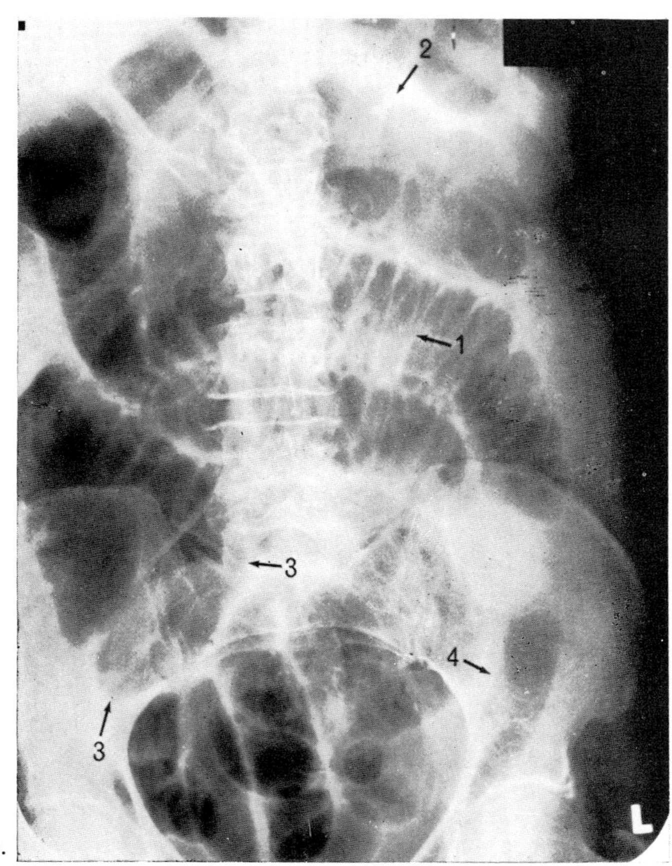

Fig. 20. Paralytic ileus.

Acute appendicitis
Fig. 21

X-RAY APPEARANCES
(Supine film)

Distended loops of bowel in the upper abdomen, displaced by a soft tissue mass in the right iliac fossa.
Faecolith in the centre of the soft tissue mass.

The distension is secondary to ileus of a loop of bowel involved in the appendix mass. In this child there was a thirty-six hour history, and at operation the appendix had perforated. See note in legend of Fig. 20 under 'differential diagnosis of X-ray'.

PRESENTATION

Central abdominal pain later becoming localized to the right iliac fossa, with tenderness and rebound tenderness.
Anorexia, nausea, and occasional vomiting.
Usually constipation, but occasionally diarrhoea.
Low-grade pyrexia, which rises when perforation or peritonitis occurs.

The presentation may be atypical in the young, the old, in pregnancy and in those patients having steroid therapy.

CLINICAL DIFFERENTIAL DIAGNOSIS

In adults

Gastroenteritis.
Perforated peptic ulcer.
Acute cholecystitis.
Diverticulitis.
Crohn's disease.
Carcinoma of the caecum either by perforation or by obstruction of the appendix.
Pyelonephritis, acute cystitis.
Rupture or torsion of an ovarian cyst.
Rupture of an ectopic pregnancy.
Salpingitis or tubo-ovarian abscess.
Inflammation of Meckel's diverticulum.
Porphyria.

In children

Mesenteric adenitis (including glandular fever).
Gastroenteritis.
Acute nephritis.
Urinary infection.
Inguinal and iliac adenitis.
Torsion of the right testicle (with pain referred to the iliac fossa).
Acute inflammation of the hip.
Henoch–Schonlein purpura: Intussusception.

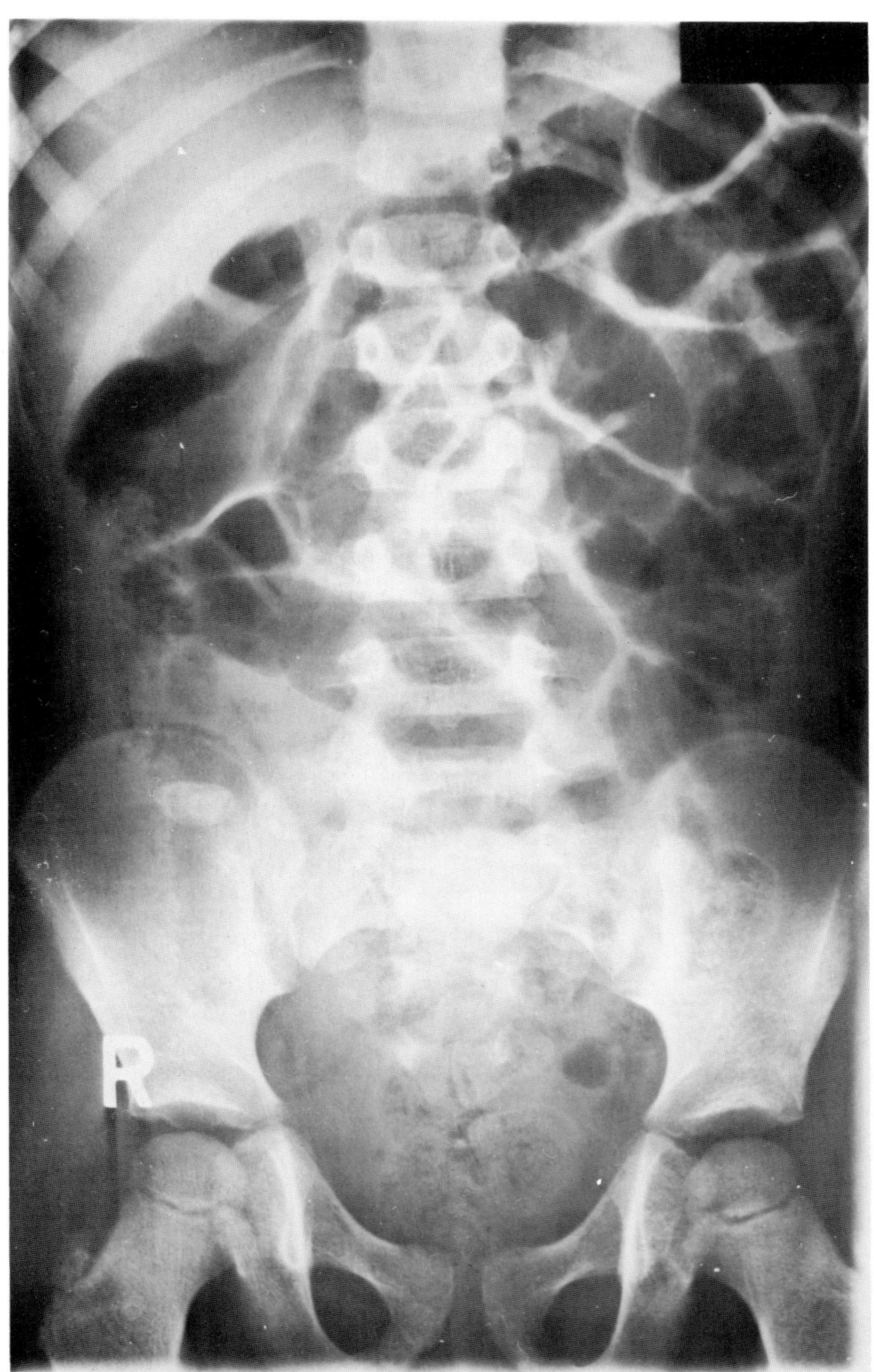

Fig. 21. Acute appendicitis.

Acute appendicitis
Fig. 22

X-RAY APPEARANCES

Two faecoliths lying in a vertically placed retro-caecal appendix.

Two gas shadows representing a segment of localized paralytic (adynamic) ileus in the region of the acutely inflamed appendix—the 'sentinel loop'.

Well-marked psoas shadows.

Other unrelated features

The left renal outline is almost triangular, a common variant of normal. Normal bladder shadow.

The 'sentinel loop' will be situated in the right iliac fossa when the appendix is in the other common positions. The presence of a faecolith on X-ray is not significant in the absence of physical signs of appendicitis. Acute appendicitis more frequently occurs without evidence of a faecolith. It is not necessary to X-ray a patient in whom a confident diagnosis of acute appendicitis can be made on clinical grounds; in the early stages most will have a normal plain abdominal X-ray.

DIFFERENTIAL DIAGNOSIS OF X-RAY

Ureteric calculus.
Calcified mesenteric lymph gland.

PRESENTATION

See legend to Fig. 21.

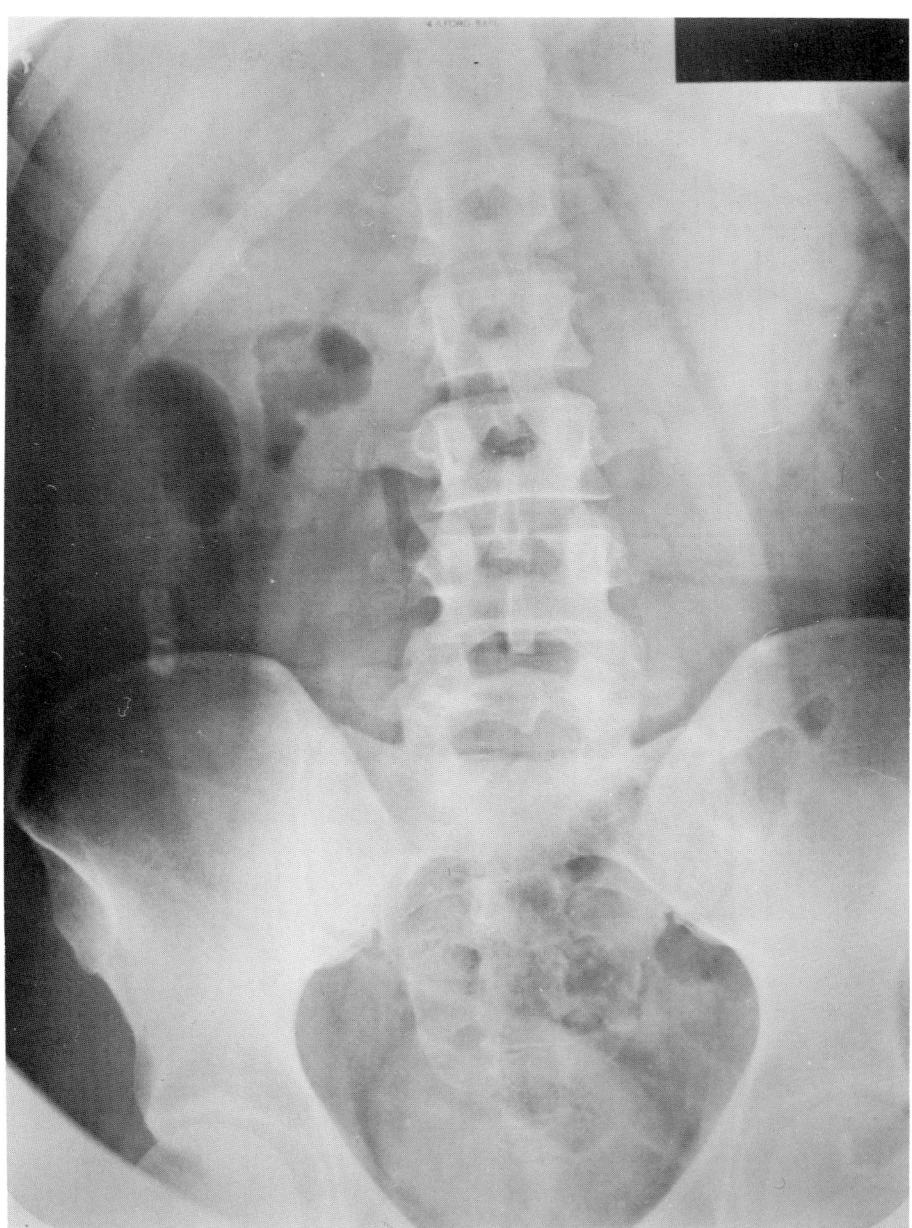

Fig. 22. Acute appendicitis.

Mechanical obstruction of small bowel Figs 23 and 24 (see also Fig. 80a and b)

X-RAY APPEARANCES

Fig. 23 (supine film)

Distended loops of small bowel, mainly in the left half of the abdomen.
Colostomy site in the left iliac fossa, arrowed.
Gas-filled loop of bowel, probably ileum, overlying the granular appearance of the caecal contents.
Absence of air in the pelvis. This is partly due to the defunctioning nature of the colostomy and partly to the level of the obstruction. In this patient a loop of ileum had prolapsed and become obstructed in the space lateral to the colostomy.

Fig. 24 (supine film)

Distended long jejunal loop in the left upper quadrant with both ends of the loop tapering to the same point.
Absence of other distended bowel.

Unrelated features

Clear psoas and right renal outlines and a calcified mesenteric gland.

This patient had a volvulus (closed loop) of jejunum around a peritoneal band.

DIFFERENTIAL DIAGNOSIS OF X-RAY

Fig. 23

Mechanical obstruction of the colon.
Peritonitis causing paralytic ileus.

Fig. 24

Obstruction due to internal hernia.
Post-gastrectomy obstruction, when the loop is usually central in position.

High jejunal obstruction may present without gaseous dilatation on X-ray because early and profuse vomiting has emptied the loops. This is the reason for the absence of distended jejunum proximal to the volvulus in Fig. 24. If air in distended small bowel becomes trapped between the valvulae conniventes it may produce the 'string of beads' sign on X-ray.

PRESENTATION

Colicky central abdominal pain.
Vomiting. The more proximal the obstruction the earlier and more profuse the vomiting.
Central distension, sometimes with visible 'ladder pattern' peristalsis, and hyperactive bowel sounds.
Localized tenderness or rebound tenderness suggests strangulation of bowel.

CLINICAL DIFFERENTIAL DIAGNOSIS

Perforation of a viscus.
Acute exacerbation of a peptic ulcer.
Acute pancreatitis.
Acute cholecystitis.
Biliary or ureteric colic.
Mesenteric vascular accident.
Myocardial infarction.

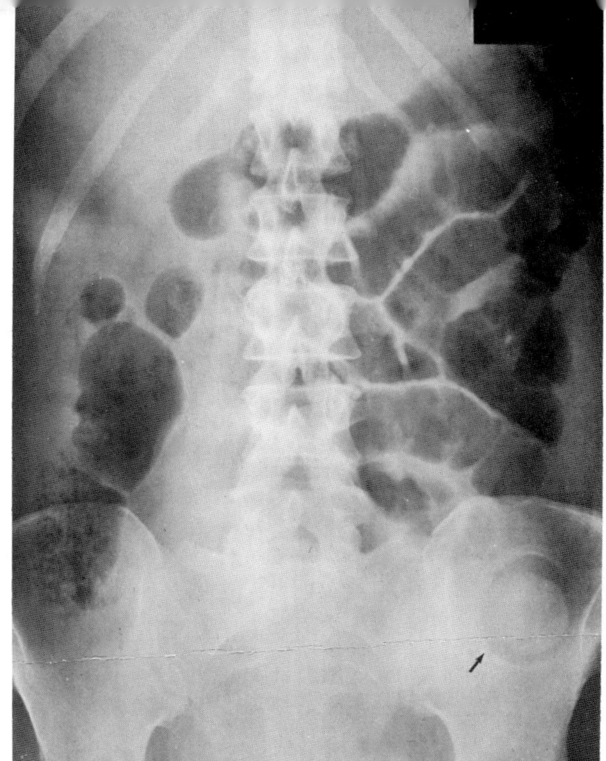

Fig. 23. Mechanical obstruction of small bowel.

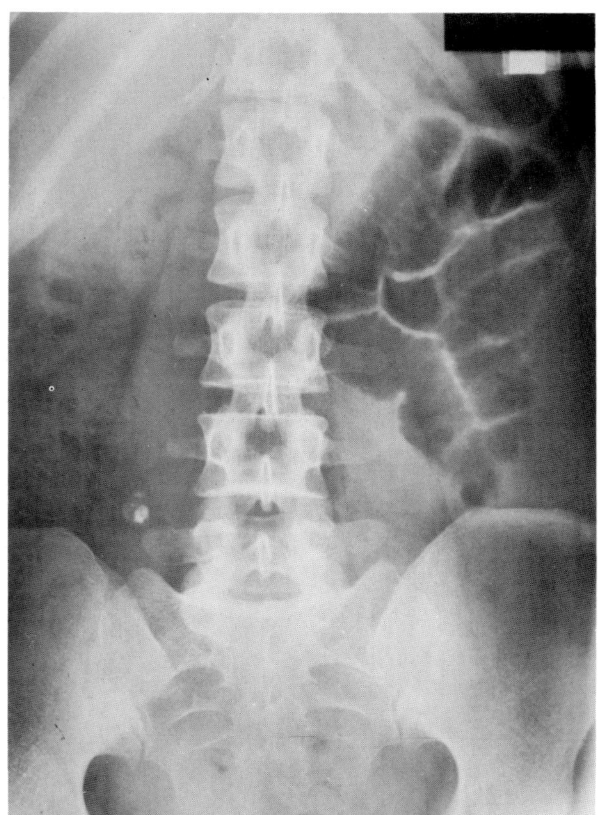

Fig. 24. Mechanical obstruction of small bowel.

Gas cysts of the small intestine
Constipation and gas cysts of colon

X-RAY APPEARANCES

Fig. 25a

Central translucent area with multiple rounded ring opacities overlying one another. Later barium studies confirmed these as ileal gas cysts. Gas cysts may also occur in the large bowel.

Faecal accumulation in the large bowel. The right colon contains semi-solid faeces showing the typical granular appearance and in the left colon there are more discrete masses of solid faeces outlined by gas between the haustral folds.

Fig. 25b

Multiple close-packed round or oval translucencies overlying one another in the line of the descending colon. These gas cysts vary in size from 0.5 to 2.0 cm. The diagnosis was confirmed on later barium studies. Normal gastric and right colon gas outlines.

PRESENTATION AND CLINICAL DIFFERENTIAL DIAGNOSIS

Gas cysts may be symptomless but are usually demonstrated radiologically in a patient undergoing investigation for diarrhoea or the passage of mucus per rectum.

Rupture of a gas cyst produces pneumoperitoneum which is unaccompanied by signs of peritonitis, and again is sometimes noticed incidentally on a chest or abdominal film.

The cysts may be seen submucosally at sigmoidoscopy.

(a)

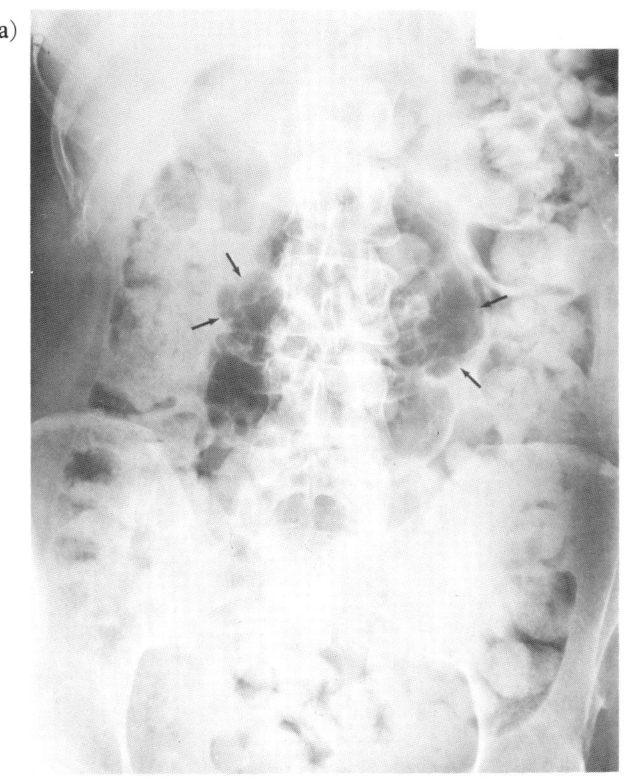

(b)

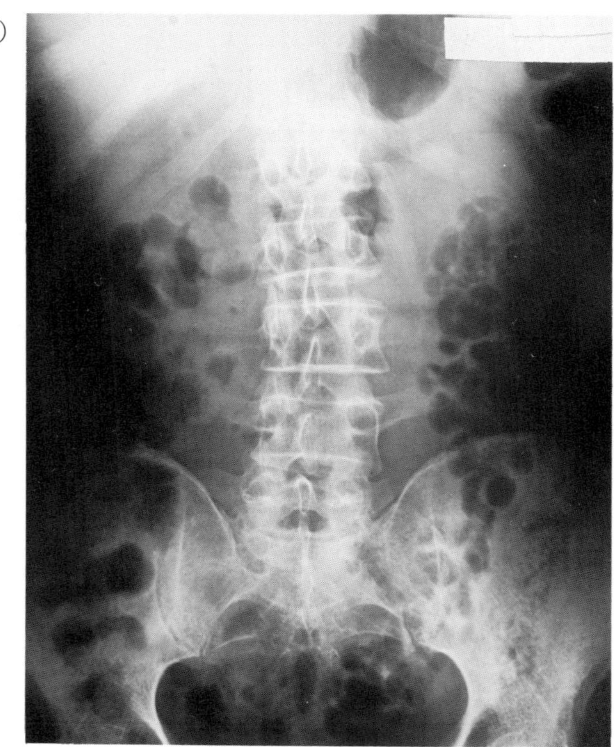

Fig. 25.a, Gas cysts of the small intestine. **b,** Gas cysts of the colon and constipation.

Mechanical obstruction of large bowel (closed loop) Fig. 26a and b

X-RAY APPEARANCES

Fig. 26a: supine film

Gross gaseous distension of the colon down to the descending-sigmoid junction, arrowed.

Absence of rectal gas.

Typical haustral pattern of the left half of the transverse colon, arrowed.

Enormous caecum and relative absence of small intestinal distension (due to a competent ileocaecal valve), signifying a closed loop obstruction.

Fig. 26b: erect film

Fluid levels in the dilated caecum, arrowed (1), and colon.

Fluid levels in slightly distended loops of small bowel, arrowed (2).

Opaque appearance of the lower half of the film due to fluid bowel contents.

Left flank stripe, arrowed (3). The proximity of the distended bowel to the flank stripe suggests that there is little intraperitoneal fluid.

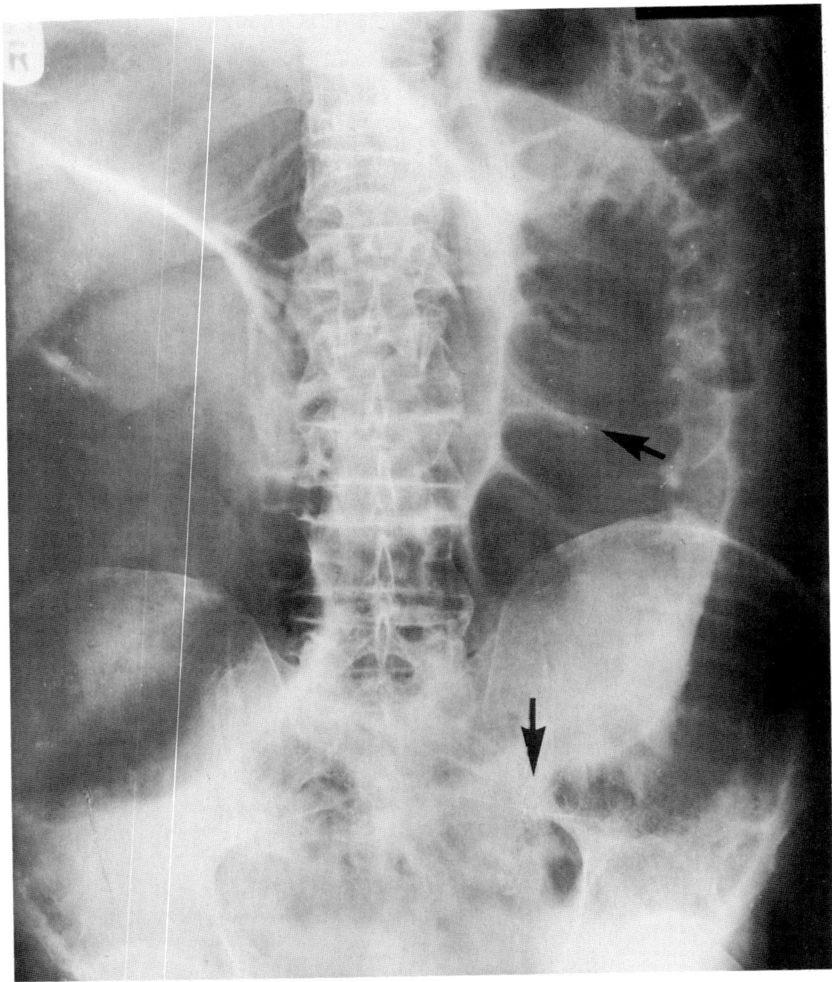

Fig. 26a (supine). Mechanical obstruction of large bowel. (Closed loop).

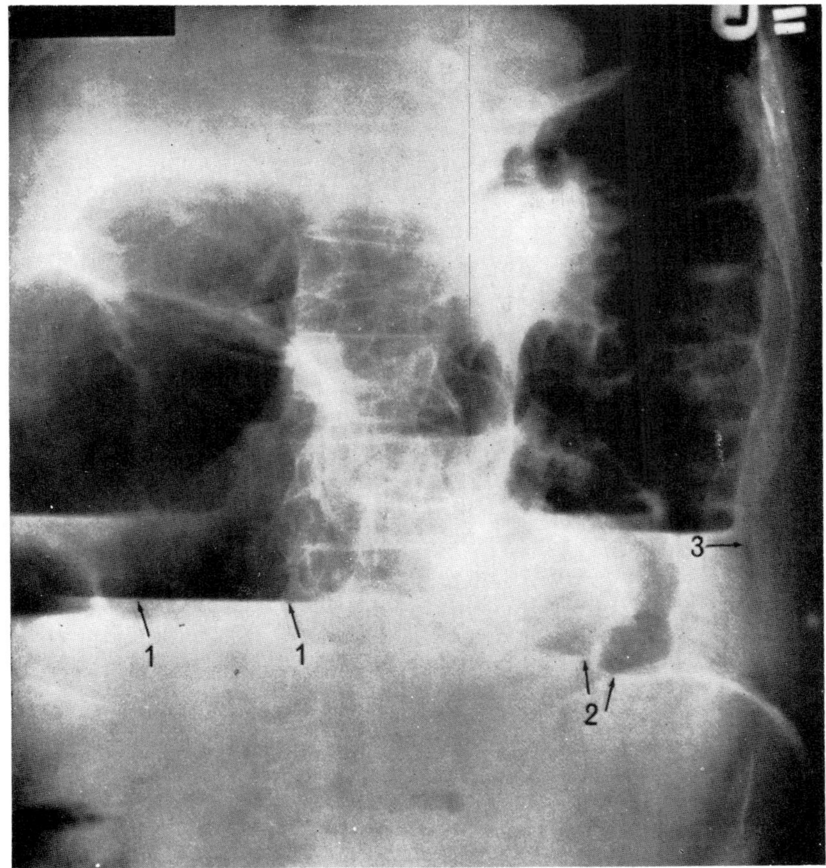

Fig. 26b (erect). Mechanical obstruction of large bowel. (Closed loop).

DIFFERENTIAL DIAGNOSIS OF X-RAY

Fig. 26a

Caecal or sigmoid volvulus.

Fig. 26b

Toxic dilatation of the colon in ulcerative colitis. Hirschsprung's disease in a child (see Fig. 78).

A barium enema or colonoscopic examination performed as an emergency procedure will demonstrate the site of the obstruction, and usually its cause.

PRESENTATION

Constipation.
Colicky abdominal pain, soon becoming continuous.
Minimal, late vomiting.
Distension, most marked in the flanks, with resonance.
Tenderness over the distended caecum is a sign suggesting imminent perforation.

CLINICAL DIFFERENTIAL DIAGNOSIS

Carcinoma or inflammatory stricture of the left colon.
Volvulus of the caecum or sigmoid colon.
Faecal impaction.
Distal small bowel obstruction.
Toxic dilatation of the colon.

Mechanical obstruction of large bowel (with incompetent ileocaecal valve) Fig. 27

X-RAY APPEARANCES (Erect film)

Gaseous distension of the transverse colon, and hepatic and splenic flexures, with fluid levels.
Multiple fluid levels in distended loops of small intestine (cf. Fig. 80b).
Absence of air in the caecum.
Absence of air in the sigmoid colon and rectum.
Diffuse 'ground glass' appearance suggesting ascites.

The caecum is not outlined by gas because it contains fluid faeces; on a supine film its site would be seen. The sigmoid colon is similarly filled with fluid proximal to an obstructing carcinoma of the recto-sigmoid junction.

The different heights of the fluid levels in the transverse colon are caused by peristalsis on either side of the fluid-filled loop. In paralytic (adynamic) ileus the fluid levels would often be at the same height on each side of the loop, although this is not a reliable differentiating sign.

DIFFERENTIAL DIAGNOSIS OF X-RAY

This appearance could only represent mechanical obstruction of the distal large bowel (see legend to Fig. 20 describing the X-ray appearances following the administration of an enema).

PRESENTATION AND CLINICAL DIFFERENTIAL DIAGNOSIS

See legends to Fig. 26.

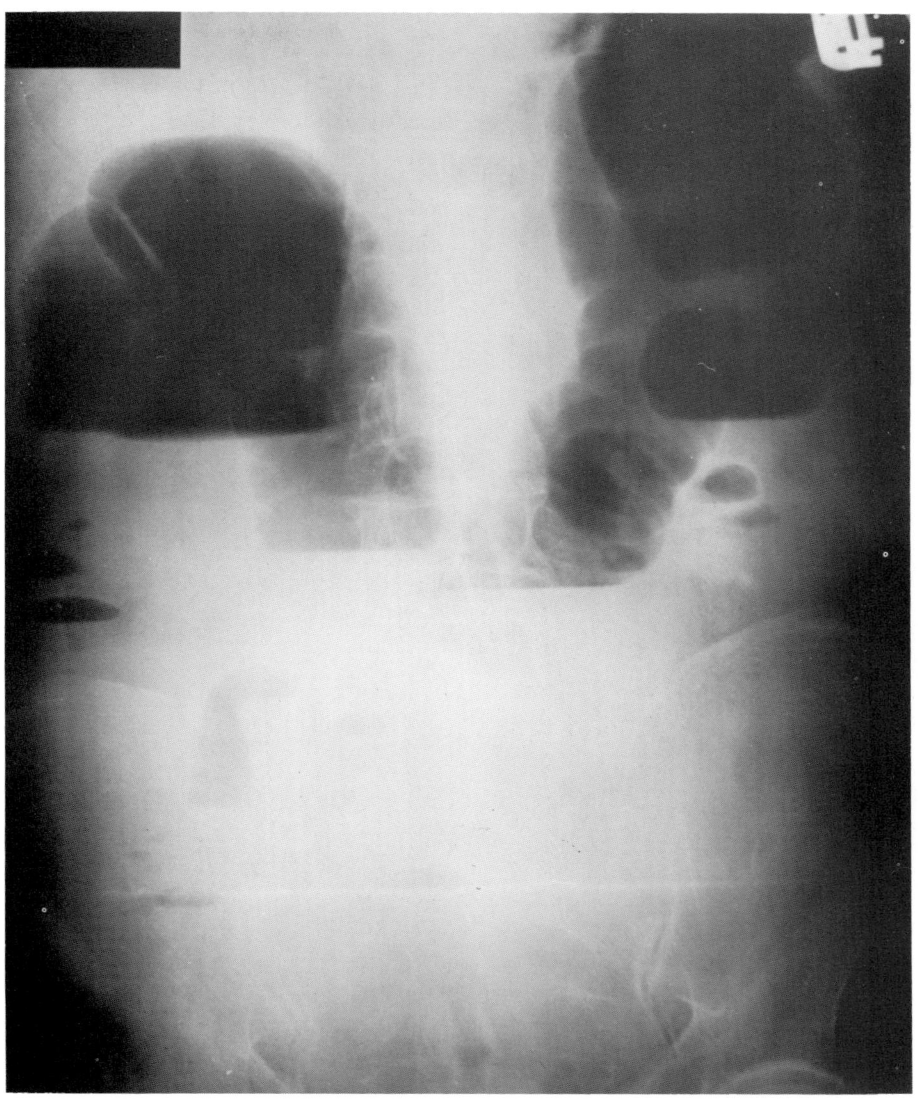

Fig. 27. Mechanical obstruction of large bowel (with incompetent ileo-caecal valve).

Intestinal pseudo-obstruction
Fig. 28

X-RAY APPEARANCES

(Supine film)

Grossly distended large bowel with, centrally, a loop of transverse colon overlying the liver shadow, see Fig. 8.
Distended small bowel loops with clear mucosal pattern.
Gas and fluid in the stomach fundus.
Vertebral osteoporosis.

These appearances are not specific and cannot be differentiated from those produced by mechanical obstruction. The patient was a 74-year-old man with a one week history of increasing constipation and painless distension. Extensive investigation including eventually a laparotomy failed to demonstrate an organic obstruction. He eventually made a complete recovery. This form of adynamic ileus occurs in diabetic and uraemic patients and also in some patients having medication with anticholinergic, anti-depressant or anti-Parkinsonian drugs. It also occurs in patients with a high alcoholic intake. It may be aggravated by the hypokalaemia which may follow prolonged diuretic usage. In the past it has been known as Ogilvie's syndrome.

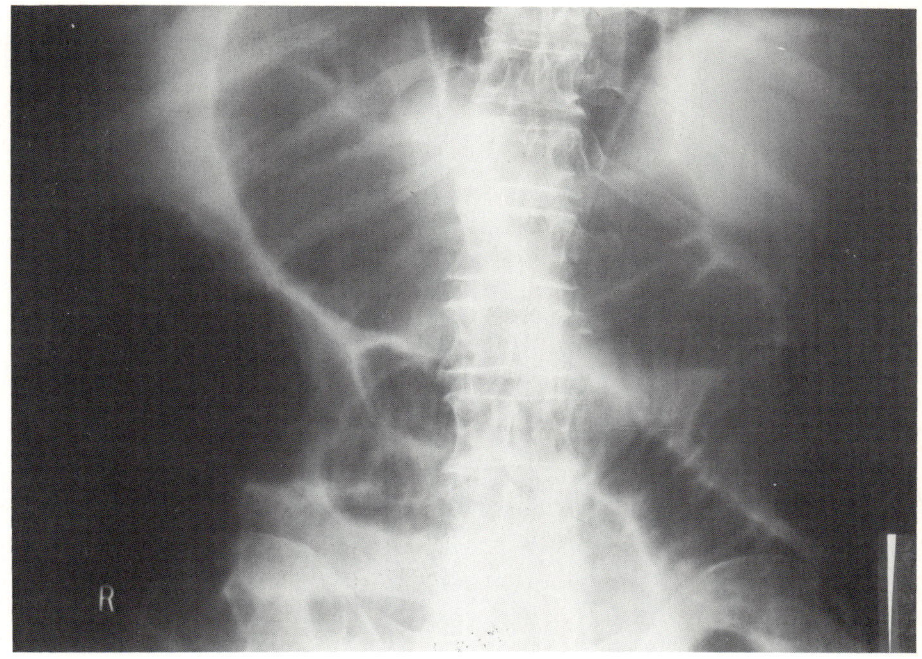

Fig. 28. Intestinal pseudo-obstruction.

Perforation of the colon: stercoral ulceration
Fig. 29

X-RAY APPEARANCES
(Supine film)

Faecal accumulation in the hepatic flexure.
The pattern of translucency around and overlying the mass suggests the presence of gas in the bowel wall (cf. Fig. 79: necrotizing enterocolitis).
Free gas in the subhepatic space, arrowed.
Caecal gas.
Faeces in the descending colon.
Calcification opposite the left second lumbar transverse process, probably in the splenic artery.
Calcification in the costal cartilages.

This patient had a neoplastic stricture of the transverse colon. Stercoral ulceration led to perforation and peritonitis. Perforation of the colon more typically leads to obvious pneumoperitoneum. Gas in the bowel wall is an uncommon finding.

PRESENTATION AND CLINICAL DIFFERENTIAL DIAGNOSIS

See legend to Figs 5 and 26.

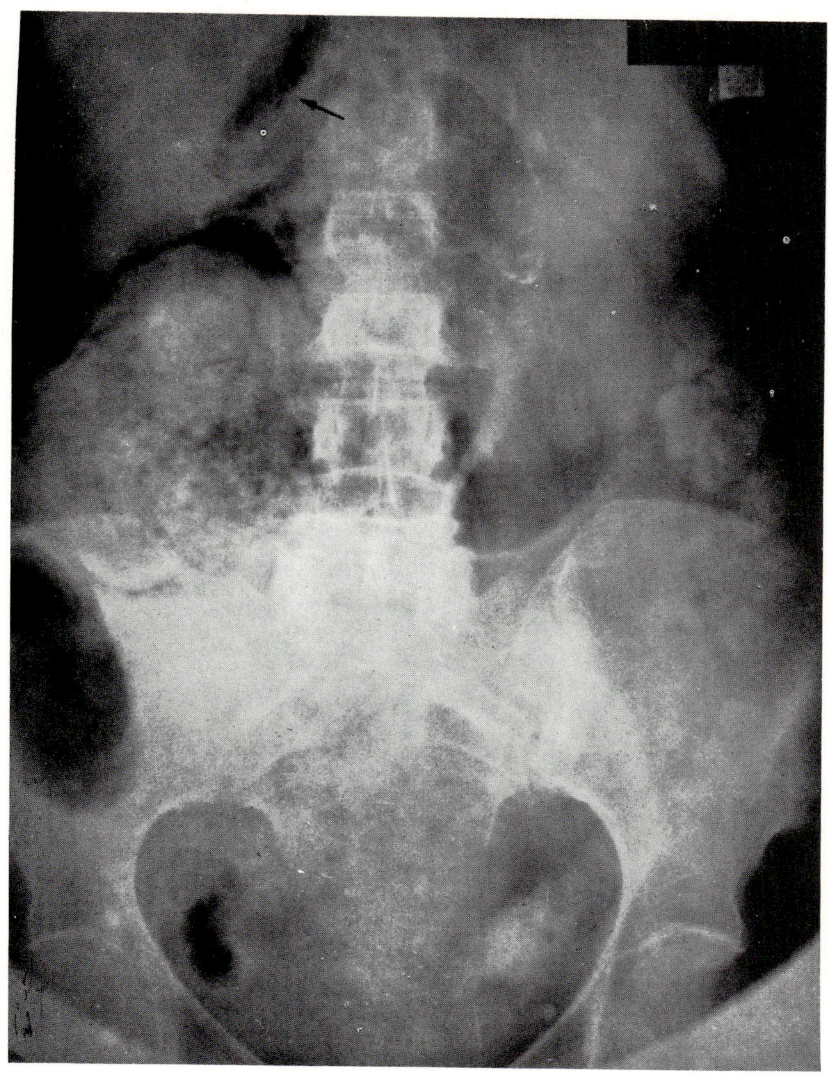

Fig. 29. Perforation of the colon. Stercoral ulceration.

Extraperitoneal perforation of the rectum
Fig. 30

X-RAY APPEARANCES

Gas in the tissue planes of the right thigh and buttock with associated soft tissue swelling. This is probably responsible for the abduction of the hip.

Residual contrast medium in the rectum and the appendix, following a barium enema.

The multiple horizontal lines across the pelvis are artefacts.

At the barium enema examination four days previously this patient was shown to have a polyp in the upper rectum. Extraperitoneal perforation occurred during biopsy.

DIFFERENTIAL DIAGNOSIS OF X-RAY

Gas gangrene.
Surgical emphysema.

PRESENTATION

Painful swelling of the thigh.
Rectal bleeding.
Pyrexia and toxaemia.

CLINICAL DIFFERENTIAL DIAGNOSIS

Endoscopic perforation of the bowel.
Impalement injury of the rectum.
Infection with gas-producing organisms.

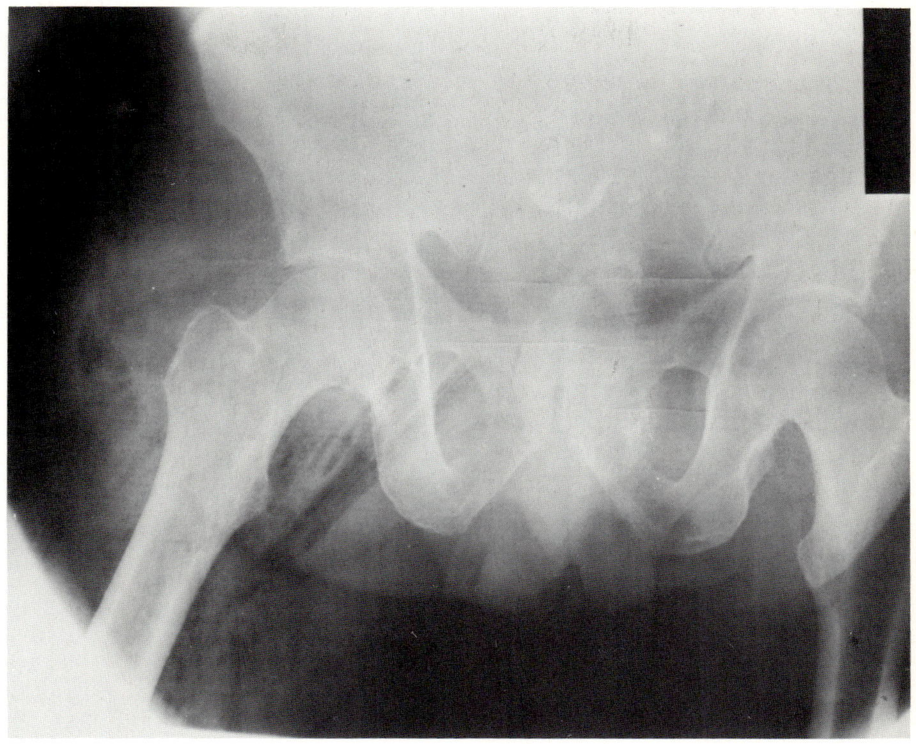

Fig. 30. Extraperitoneal perforation of the rectum.

Sigmoid volvulus
Fig. 31

X-RAY APPEARANCES
(Supine film)

Characteristic grossly-distended loop of sigmoid colon lacking any haustral markings.
Ascending and transverse colon with haustral markings, on the right of the abdomen.

The characteristic feature is the presence of the greatly dilated loop of sigmoid colon forming the so-called 'bent inner tube' or 'omega loop' sign, with the convexity of the loop lying away from the site of volvulus.

DIFFERENTIAL DIAGNOSIS OF X-RAY

Large bowel obstruction (cf. Figs 26 and 27).
Caecal volvulus.

A sigmoidoscopic or barium enema examination will confirm the diagnosis. The film taken erect of a patient with a sigmoid volvulus may show large fluid levels and must be differentiated from pneumoperitoneum with free intraperitoneal fluid (cf. Fig. 7).

PRESENTATION

In Europe the patient is often an elderly mentally handicapped male.
Constipation.
Gross, resonant, abdominal distension.
Colicky pain.

The greatest incidence of sigmoid volvulus is in the sixth and seventh decades. It is commoner in Eastern Europe and parts of Africa and Asia where high residue in the diet is thought to predispose to the condition.

CLINICAL DIFFERENTIAL DIAGNOSIS

See legend to Fig. 26.

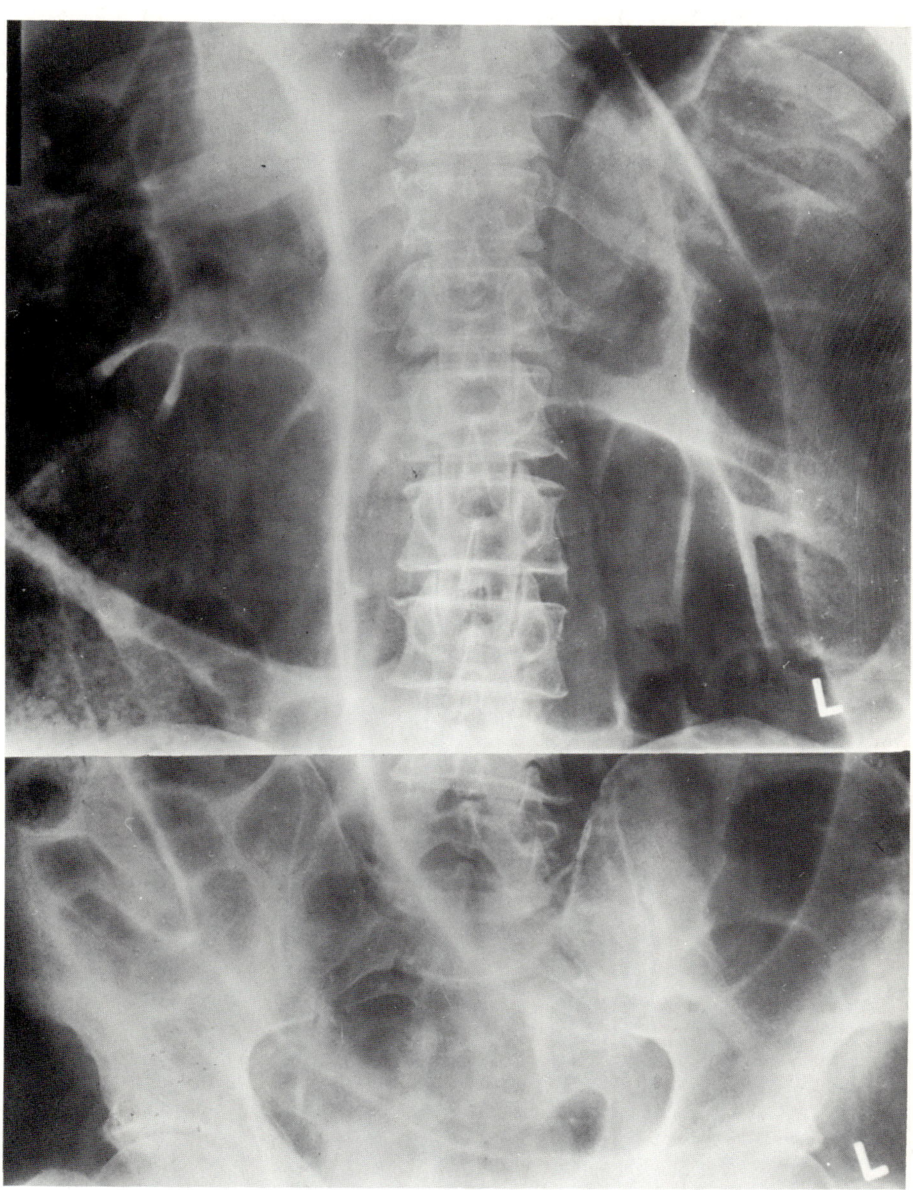

Fig. 31. Sigmoid volvulus.

Caecal volvulus
Fig. 32

X-RAY APPEARANCES

A large gas-fluid level within the colon in the left upper quadrant.
Displaced gastric gas bubble.
Absence of bowel gas in the right side of the abdomen.
Absence of gas in the rectum.

Often the volvulus is associated with an abnormal mesentery of the caecum, which allows the loop to rotate and displace to an abnormal position. It may occur in pregnancy and in the puerperium, when diagnosis may be more difficult.

The appearances are characteristic of a closed loop of large bowel which was proved at laparotomy to be a caecal volvulus.

DIFFERENTIAL DIAGNOSIS OF X-RAY

Volvulus of stomach.
Toxic megacolon.
Acute gastric dilatation.
Sigmoid volvulus (see Fig. 31).

PRESENTATION

Abdominal pain.
Gross resonant distension.
Constipation.
Late vomiting (may be preceded by similar, less severe episodes).

CLINICAL DIFFERENTIAL DIAGNOSIS

Large intestinal obstruction from any cause.
Sigmoid volvulus.
Acute gastric dilatation.

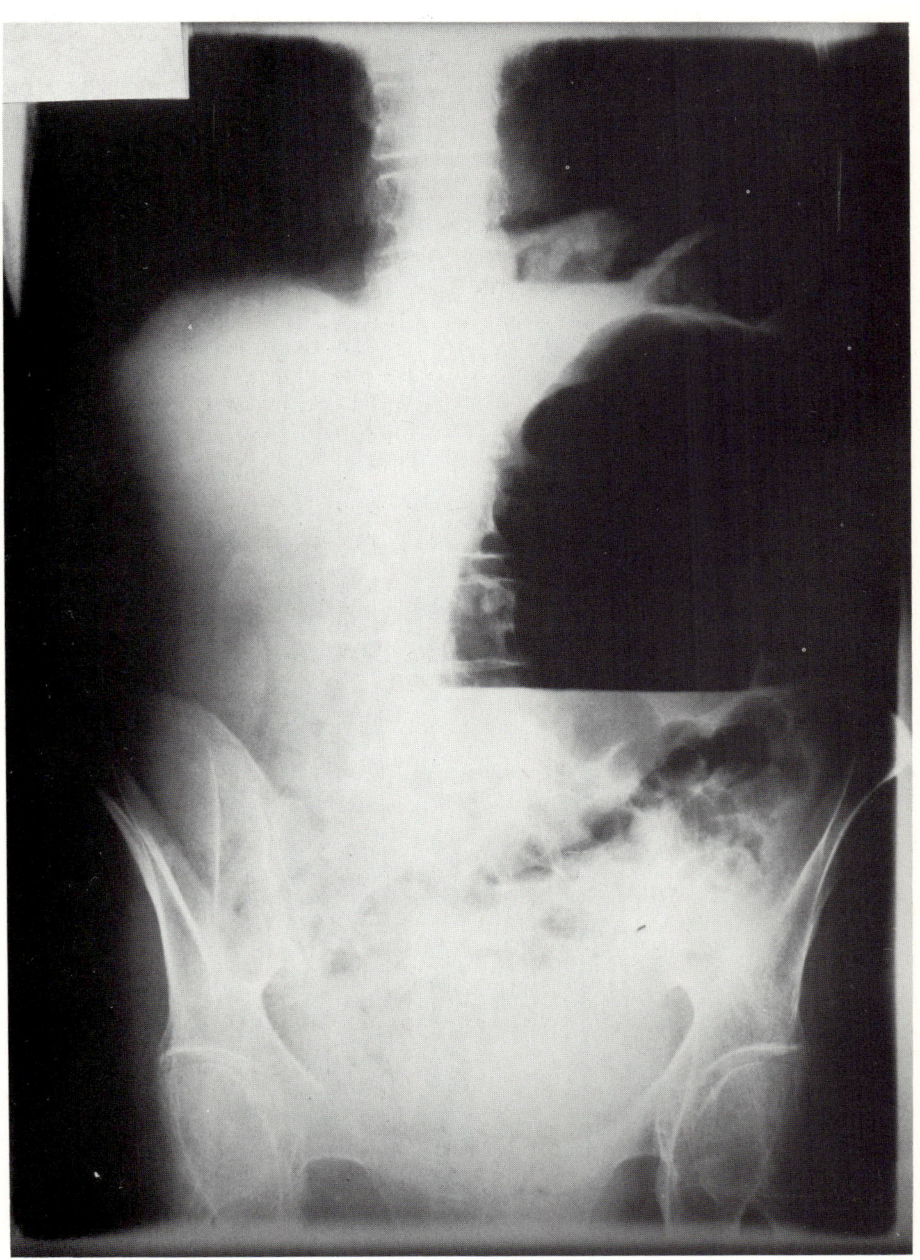

Fig. 32. Caecal volvulus.

Acute toxic dilatation of the colon: ulcerative colitis
Fig. 33

X-RAY APPEARANCES
(Supine film)

Transverse and descending colonic distension, with absence of haustrations.
Multiple rounded soft-tissue shadows projecting into the lumen of the colon.
Granular appearance of the faecal content of the right colon.
The wall of the descending colon (arrowed) appears thickened and straight due to oedema.

The shadows projecting into the lumen are islands of oedematous and haemorrhagic mucosa (pseudo-polypi) between extensive areas of ulceration. The transverse colon is the most commonly affected segment.

DIFFERENTIAL DIAGNOSIS OF X-RAY

Multiple colonic polyposis with distal obstruction.
Ischaemic colitis.

PRESENTATION

This condition usually presents as acute progression of known ulcerative colitis, with abdominal distension, lessening of the diarrhoea, colicky pains, generalized or localized tenderness and pyrexia in an obviously ill patient.
In an initial acute attack of ulcerative colitis, or sometimes during the progression of known disease, the clinical features may not suggest this serious complication, particularly when the patient is being treated with steroids. Straight X-ray of the abdomen will be diagnostic and if repeated at intervals may demonstrate increasing dilatation, or an unsuspected perforation, both of which are indications for surgical intervention.

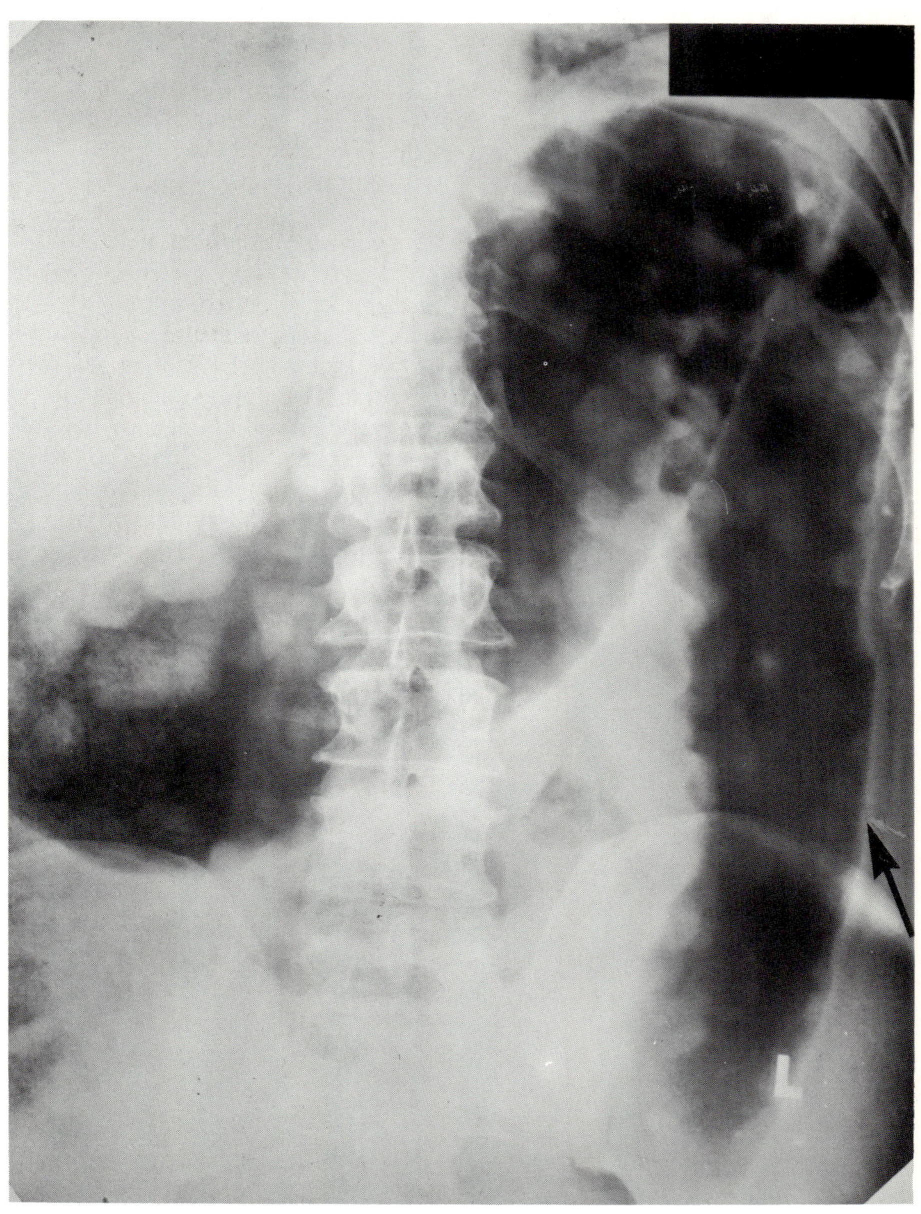

Fig. 33. Acute toxic dilatation of the colon.

Chronic ulcerative colitis
Fig. 34

X-RAY APPEARANCES
(Supine film)

Gas outlining a tubular, featureless 'hose-pipe' from the mid-transverse to the distal descending and sigmoid colon.

Absence of haustral marking with shortening and straightening of the loops.

Normal appearances in the right, unaffected half of the colon.

Pseudo-polypi or ulceration are not seen in this chronic state of the disease (see Fig. 33).

DIFFERENTIAL DIAGNOSIS OF X-RAY

Late stage (after healing) of ischaemic colitis.

In the descending colon this featureless appearance may sometimes be normal. It is not normal in the transverse colon.

PRESENTATION AND CLINICAL FEATURES

Chronic diarrhoea, with exacerbations.

Passage of slime and blood per rectum.

Colicky or continuous left-sided abdominal pain.

The patient may present with mild bowel symptoms or a secondary manifestation of ulcerative colitis such as pyoderma gangrenosum, arthropathy or liver disease. The X-ray appearances may then be helpful in making the diagnosis and should be supported by barium studies and colonoscopy with biopsy. The possibility of carcinoma developing in long-standing colitis must be kept in mind.

CLINICAL DIFFERENTIAL DIAGNOSIS

Carcinoma of rectum or colon.

Chronic infective or parasitic diarrhoea.

Crohn's disease of the colon.

Ischaemic colitis.

Small bowel or pancreatic diarrhoea.

Gastro-colic fistula.

Diverticulitis.

Irritable colon.

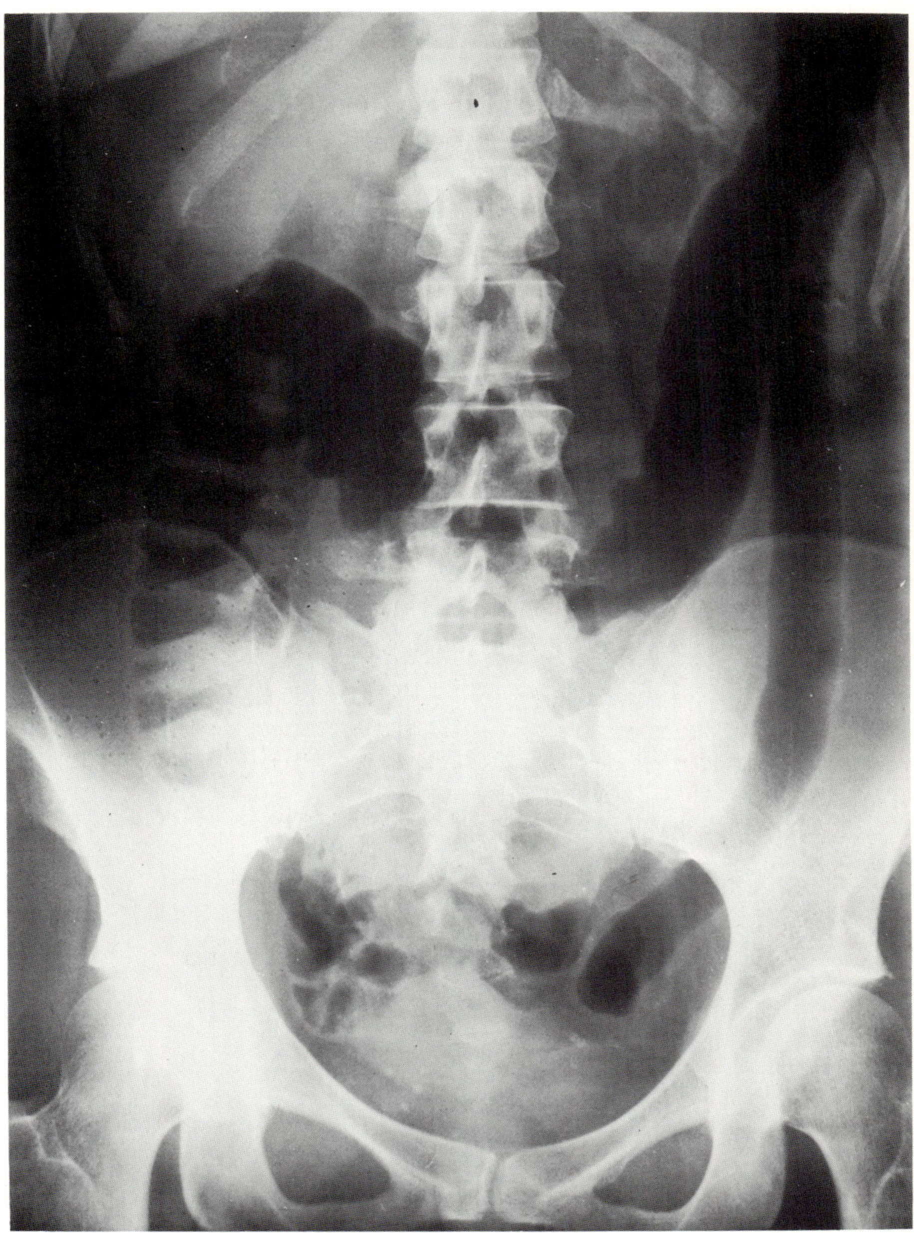

Fig. 34. Chronic ulcerative colitis.

Ischaemic colitis
Fig. 35

X-RAY APPEARANCES
(Supine film)

Broad-based polypoid projections ('thumb-prints') into the lumen of the distal section of the transverse colon.

The change becomes less marked towards the mid-transverse colon.

Distension of the proximal colon: note the haustra.

Normal gas outline of the descending colon.

Unrelated feature

Calcified mesenteric gland.

Occlusion of a colic artery, if it does not lead to gangrene, is followed by oedema of the wall of the bowel. The commonest segment of the colon to be affected by ischaemia is, as in this patient, the splenic flexure. The enlarged mucosal folds project into the lumen producing the 'thumb-print' sign which is more usually seen on barium enema examination. 'Thumb-printing' is not always seen as clearly as in this example. A segment of bowel so affected may cause functional obstruction, which on this film is suggested by the colonic distension. The more usual appearances of ischaemic colitis are simply those of large bowel obstruction (cf. Figs 26 and 27). Similarly, occlusion of a jejunal or ileal artery by thrombosis or embolus usually produces the X-ray appearances of small bowel obstruction (see Figs 23, 24 and 80); thickening of the wall of a distended loop of bowel due to intramural haemorrhage and oedema may be seen, but thumb-printing is absent.

DIFFERENTIAL DIAGNOSIS OF X-RAY

Acute ulcerative colitis.
Crohn's disease of the colon.

PRESENTATION

Lower abdominal pain and tenderness of sudden onset.

Diarrhoea with passage of bright blood per rectum.

Vomiting.

Pyrexia.

CLINICAL DIFFERENTIAL DIAGNOSIS

Acute infective gastroenteritis.
Carcinoma of the colon.
Acute ulcerative colitis.
Acute diverticulitis of the colon.
Infarction of small intestine.
Intussusception.

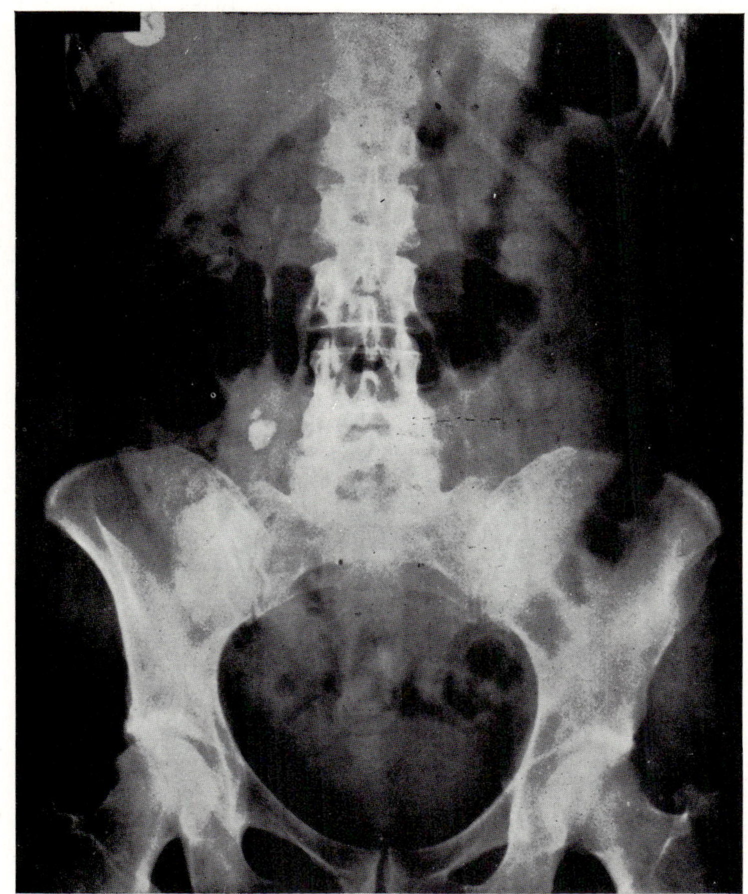

Fig. 35. Ischaemic colitis.

Superior mesenteric artery occlusion
Fig. 36

X-RAY APPEARANCES
(Supine film)

Distended loops of small intestine in the abdomen and pelvis.
Intramural gas in many of these loops. The gas is particularly well seen in the left hypochondrium where the loops overlie the soft tissue shadow produced by a fluid and gas filled stomach.

These appearances are characteristic of mesenteric infarction of some hours duration. They are similar to but more extensive than the changes which occur in the newborn suffering from necrotizing enterocolitis (Fig. 79).

PRESENTATION

Sudden acute and severe central abdominal pain.
Vomiting.
Abdominal distension.
Generalized tenderness.
Shock out of proportion to the abdominal signs.

Examination of the cardiovascular system may suggest the source of an arterial embolus e.g. a recent myocardial infarct or atrial fibrillation.

There may alternatively be evidence of generalized arterial disease which suggests that mesenteric arterial thrombosis has occurred. In a younger patient midgut volvulus secondary to congenital malrotation may be responsible.

CLINICAL DIFFERENTIAL DIAGNOSIS

See legend to Figs 23 and 24.

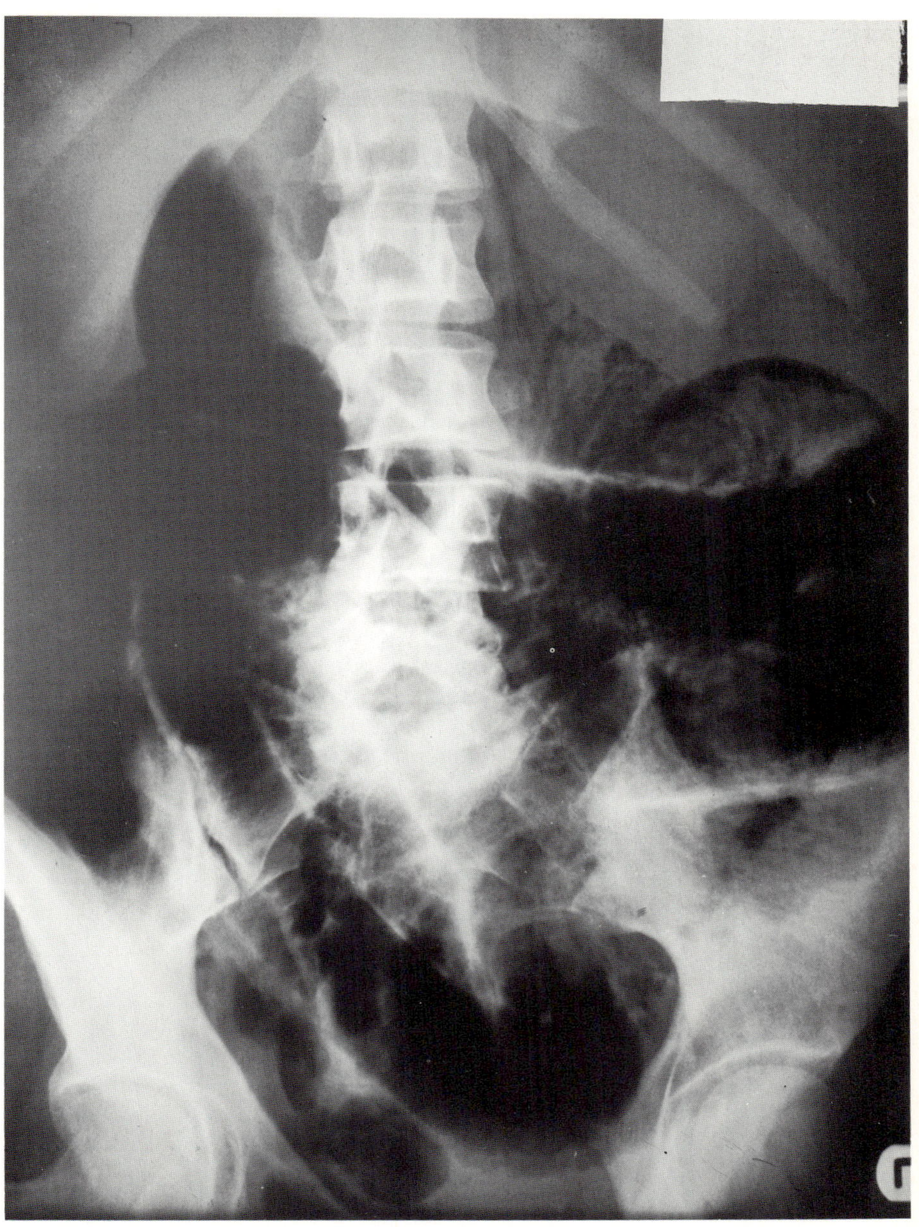

Fig. 36. Superior mesenteric artery occlusion.

Pelvic abscess
Fig. 37

X-RAY APPEARANCES
(Supine film)

Diffuse opacity in the true pelvis.
Several loops of distended small bowel 'passing into' the region of the opacity.
Distension of the proximal small bowel in the central abdomen (note mucosal folds across the whole diameter of the loops).
Scattered gas in the descending colon implying incomplete obstruction proximally.

These appearances are produced by segmental paralytic ileus of loops of bowel in contact with the abscess. The proximal bowel dilates secondarily. See also Figs 21 and 80a and b.

DIFFERENTIAL DIAGNOSIS OF X-RAY

Intestinal obstruction due to an adhesion or internal hernia.
Torsion of an ovarian cyst with adherent bowel.
Intestinal obstruction with a full bladder.

PRESENTATION

An abdominal illness of several days' duration.
Lower abdominal pain.
Vomiting.
Pyrexia.
Anorexia.
Frequency or difficulty with micturition.
Diarrhoea or constipation.
Suprapubic tenderness and/or mass.
Rectal tenderness and/or mass.
Abdominal distension.

CLINICAL DIFFERENTIAL DIAGNOSIS

The common causes of pelvic abscess are:
Perforated diverticulitis of the colon.
Appendicitis or salpingitis.
After colonic surgery this X-ray suggests an anastomotic leak.

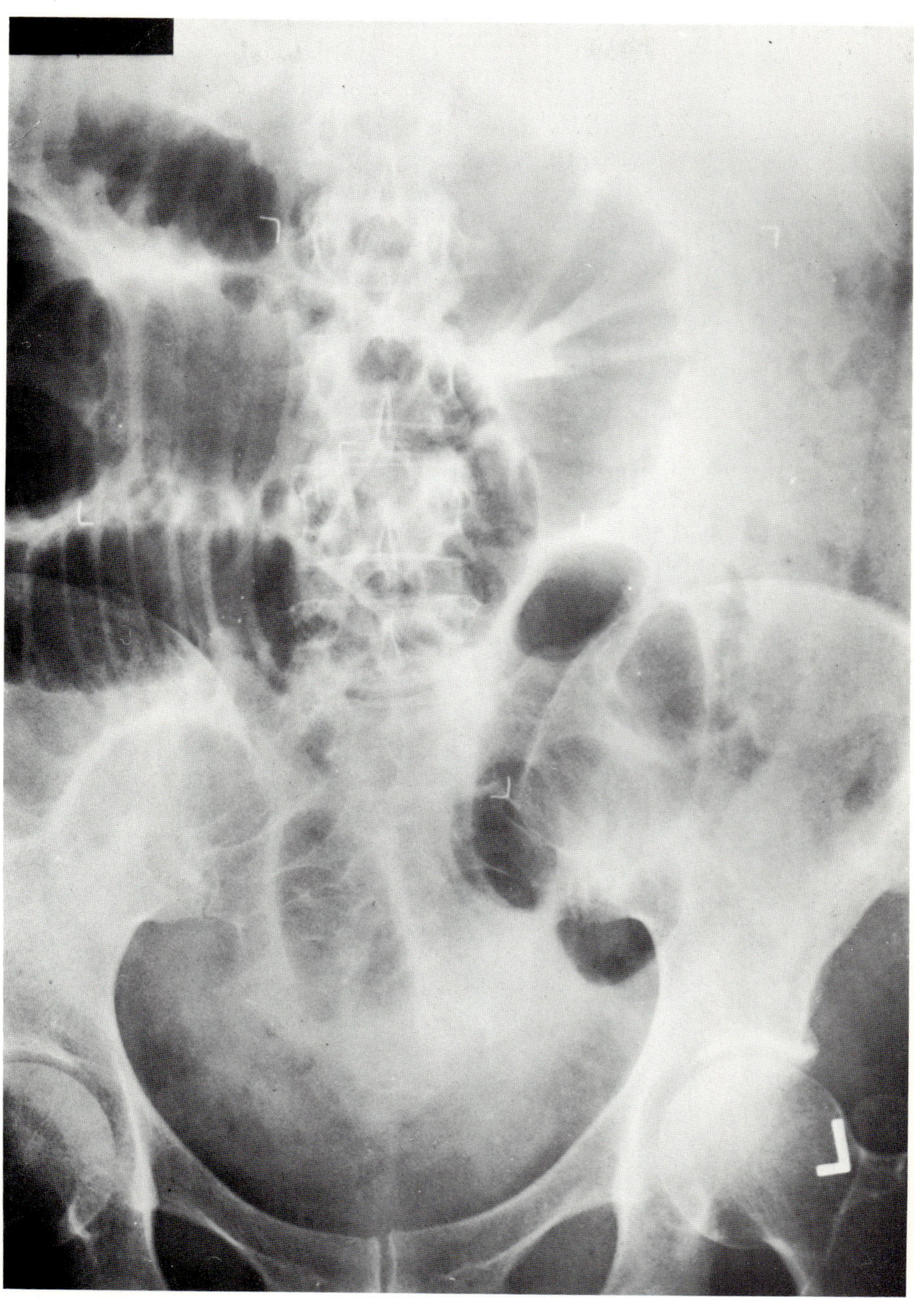

Fig. 37. Pelvic abscess.

Subphrenic abscess
Fig. 38a and b

X-RAY APPEARANCES (P.A. and lateral chest films)

Subdiaphragmatic gas bubble and fluid level on the left. On the lateral film this is seen to occupy much of the space under the dome of the diaphragm (unlike a gastric air bubble).

Obliteration of the left costophrenic angle, visible on both films. This is caused by a sympathetic pleural effusion, which is also visible in the interlobar fissure in the lateral film.

Raised and thickened left side of the diaphragm.

Collapse and consolidation of the left basal segments of the lung.

Partial resection of the left seventh rib.

Subdiaphragmatic gas on the right, without overlying lung changes. This suggests that the air was introduced at laparotomy.

Fluoroscopic examination (screening) will demonstrate absent or restricted diaphragmatic movement. If a subphrenic abscess is suspected ultrasonography is the first investigation; alternatively outlining the stomach with air or contrast medium will demonstrate gastric displacement.

DIFFERENTIAL DIAGNOSIS OF X-RAY

Any cause of free peritoneal gas (see legend to Fig. 5).

Lung abscess or empyema.

Intra-hepatic abscess (see Fig. 39).

PRESENTATION

In the post-operative period:

Poorly localized chest pain—sometimes referred to the shoulder tip.

Anorexia, malaise.

Persistent fever.

Anterior or posterior subcostal tenderness and, later, oedema.

CLINICAL DIFFERENTIAL DIAGNOSIS

Deep wound abscess.

Other intra-peritoneal abscesses (liver, para-colic).

Perinephric abscess.

Peritonitis.

Acute cholecystitis or cholangitis.

Degeneration of a malignant deposit in the liver.

Pancreatitis.

Septicaemia.

Empyema.

Pneumonia.

Lung abscess.

(a)

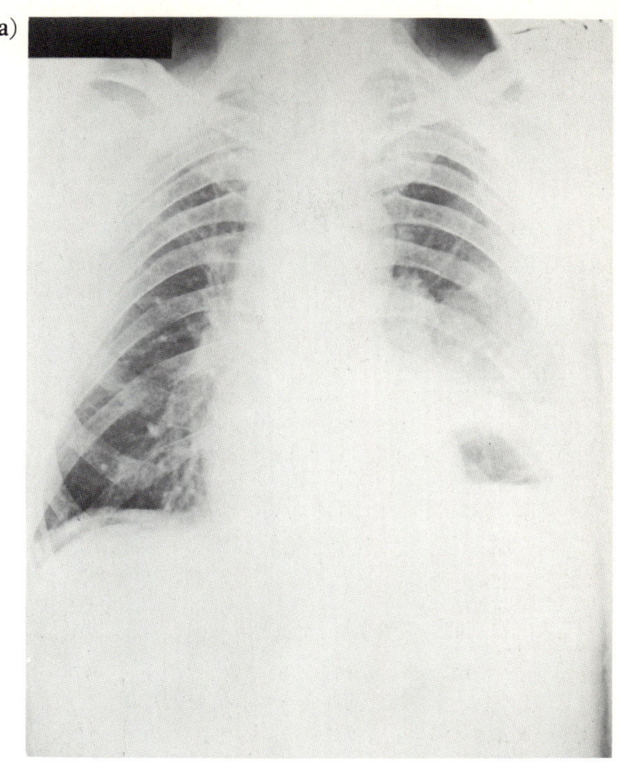

(b)

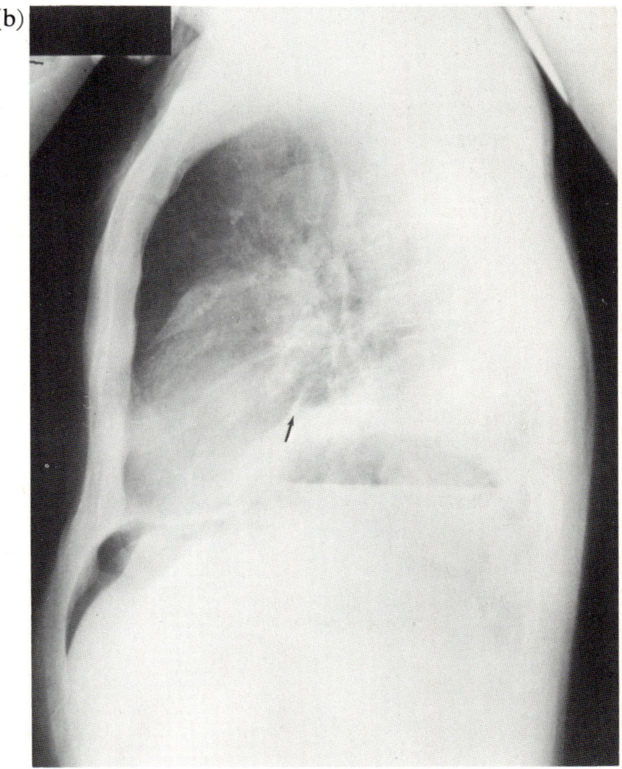

Fig. 38. Subphrenic abscess **a** P.A. **b** Lateral.

Liver abscess
Fig. 39

X-RAY APPEARANCES

Gas-fluid level in the right hypochondrium.
Raised right diaphragm.

DIFFERENTIAL DIAGNOSIS OF X-RAY

Subphrenic abscess (see Fig. 38).
Colon interposed between anterior abdominal wall and the liver (see Fig. 8).

PRESENTATION

Right upper quadrant pain.
Fever.
Jaundice.
Anorexia.
Weight loss.
Pyrexia of unknown origin.

This patient had an amoebic abscess.

CLINICAL DIFFERENTIAL DIAGNOSIS

See Fig. 38.

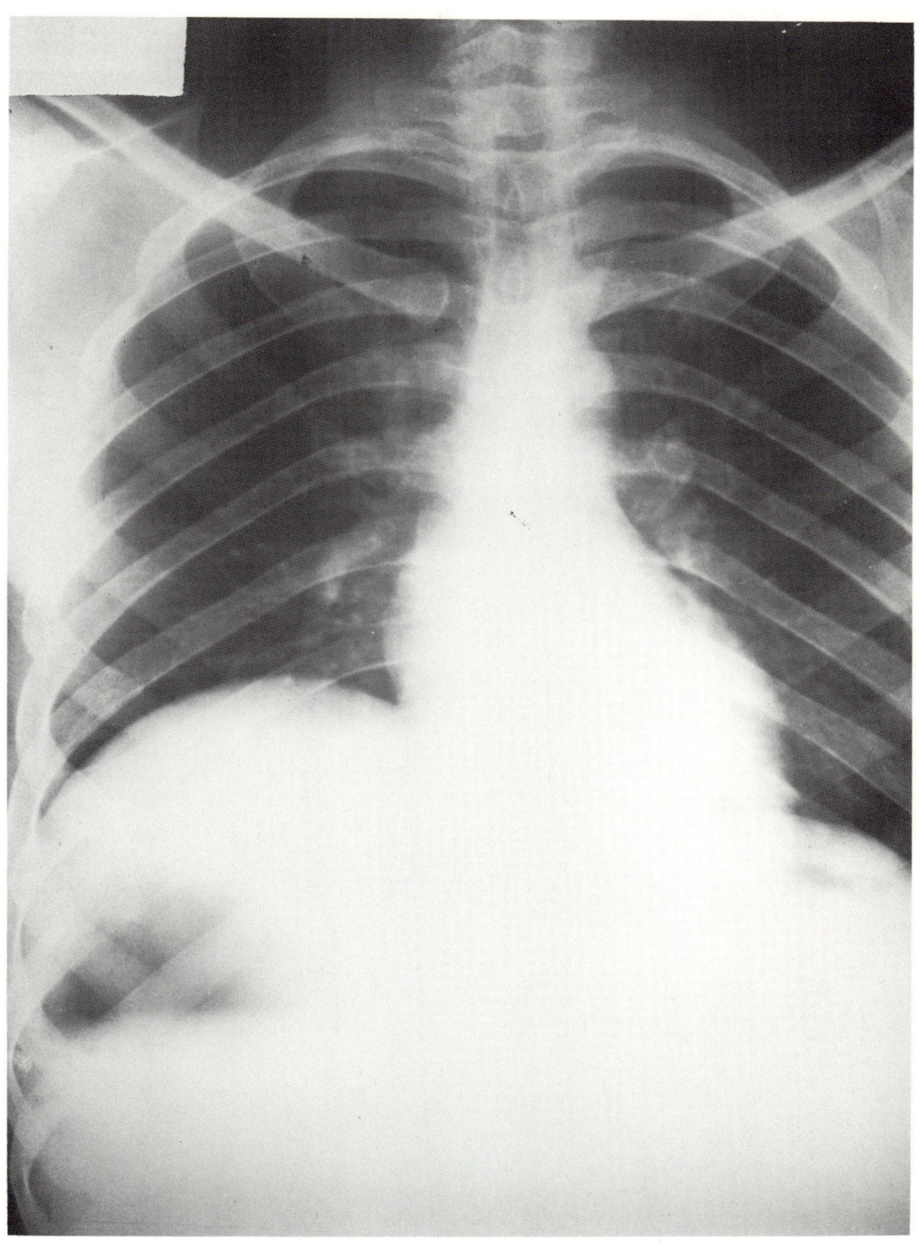

Fig. 39. Liver abscess.

Peritonitis with free fluid Fig. 40

X-RAY APPEARANCES (Supine film)

'Ground glass' appearance over the whole upper abdomen. Absence of gas shadows, excepting those in the stomach and splenic flexure.

Clear psoas shadows and renal outline.

Descending colon outlined in the left flank.

Rounded soft tissue shadow produced by the gastric fundus, arrowed. Unless the fundus is filled with gas either by nasogastric tube or a fizzy drink, or a prone film is taken, this shadow may be mistaken for an adrenal tumour.

DIFFERENTIAL DIAGNOSIS OF X-RAY

Ascites (see Fig. 41).

Haemoperitoneum.

PRESENTATION

This depends on the cause of the peritonitis.

CLINICAL DIFFERENTIAL DIAGNOSIS

Perforated peptic ulcer without free gas (see legend to Fig. 5).

Tuberculous peritonitis.

Primary peritonitis, in a child particularly.

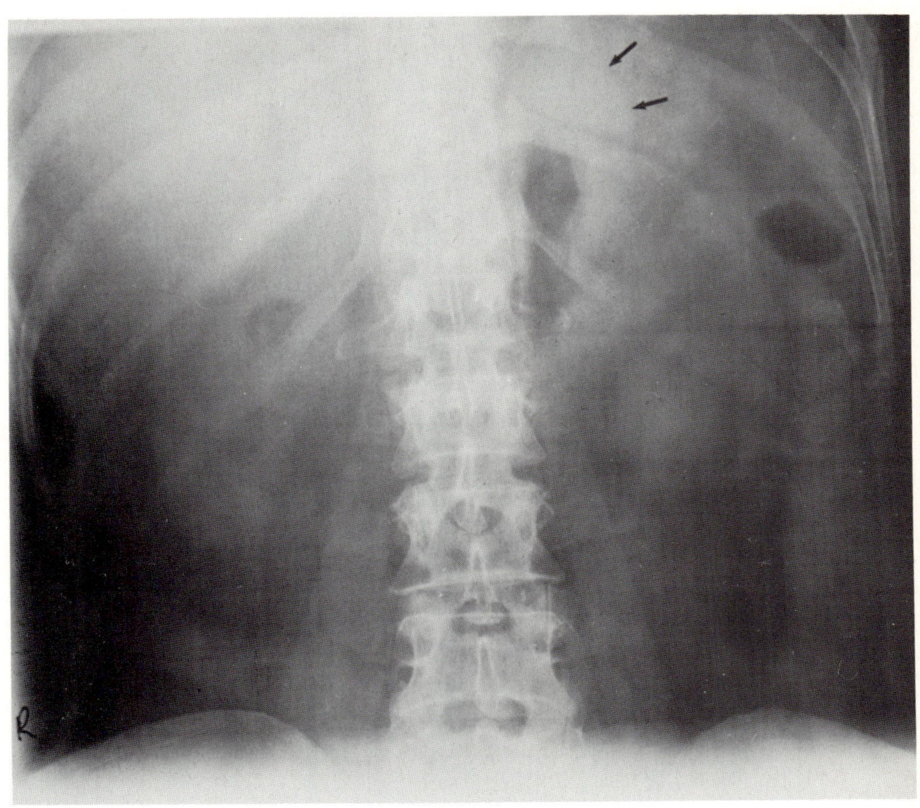

Fig. 40. Peritonitis with free fluid.

Ascites
Fig. 41

X-RAY APPEARANCES

Diffuse soft tissue opacity throughout the abdomen and pelvis.
Gas-filled stomach and first part of the duodenum.
Speckled colonic gas shadows in the right hypochondrium and right iliac fossa.
A distended small bowel loop, with valvulae conniventes, in the left central abdomen.
Bulging flanks.

This patient had gross ascites and partial small bowel obstruction secondary to a carcinoma of the ovary. Other causes of ascites include hepatic cirrhosis, cardiac failure, Budd–Chiari syndrome.

PRESENTATION

Abdominal distension.
Weight loss, anorexia.
Symptom of intestinal obstruction.

CLINICAL DIFFERENTIAL DIAGNOSIS

Large ovarian cyst.
Pregnancy.
Chronic urinary retention.
Obesity.

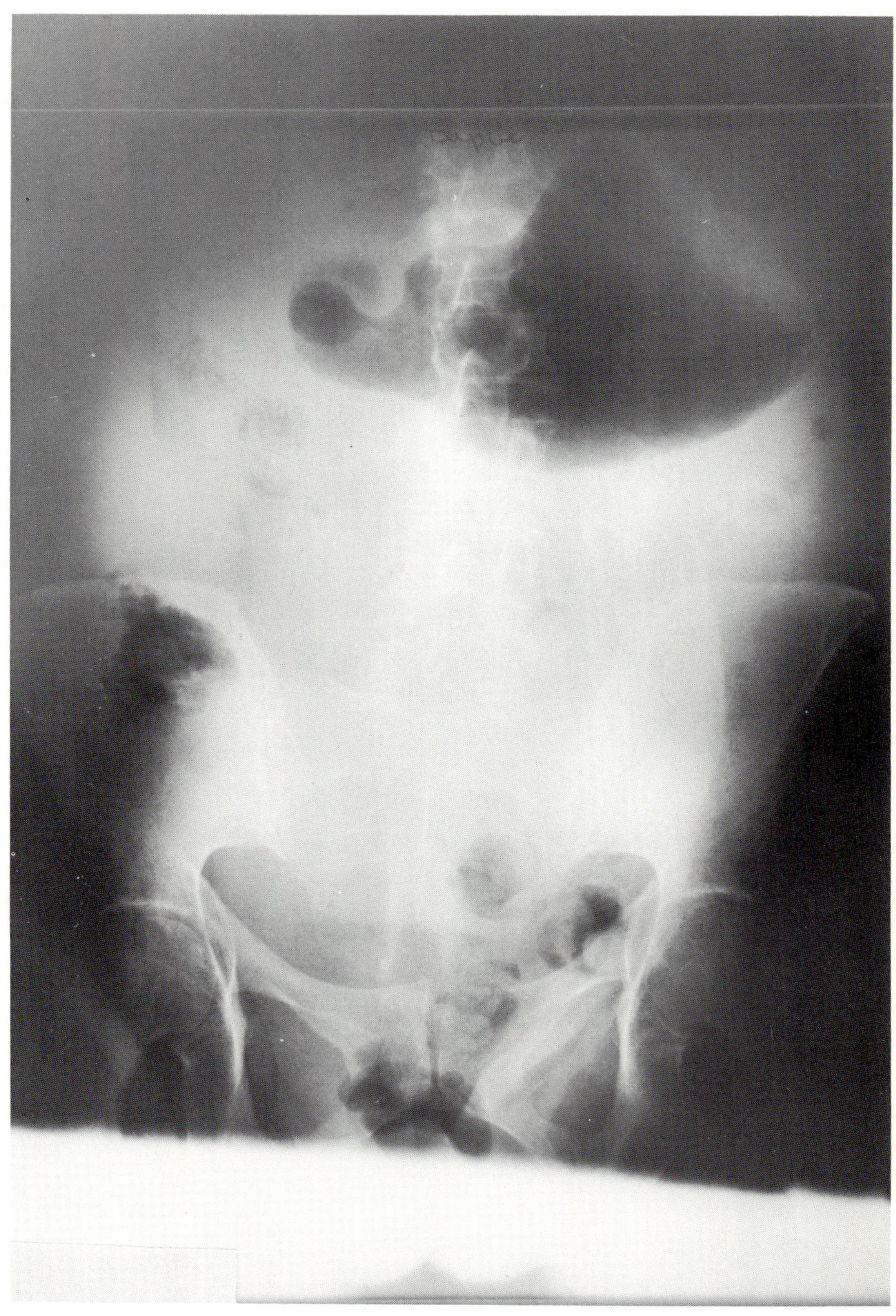

Fig. 41. Ascites.

Right basal pneumonia
Fig. 42

This film is included to stress the importance of a thorough clinical examination of the chest in every patient presenting with abdominal pain.

X-RAY APPEARANCES

The air under both sides of the diaphragm was introduced during a laparotomy at which no abnormality was found.

This X-ray, taken subsequently, suggested that the correct diagnosis was abdominal pain referred from the parietal pleura. It should be remembered that in the early stages of pneumonia physical signs in the chest may be few.

DIFFERENTIAL DIAGNOSIS OF X-RAY

All the causes of pneumoperitoneum (see legend Fig. 5) in the presence of basal consolidation.

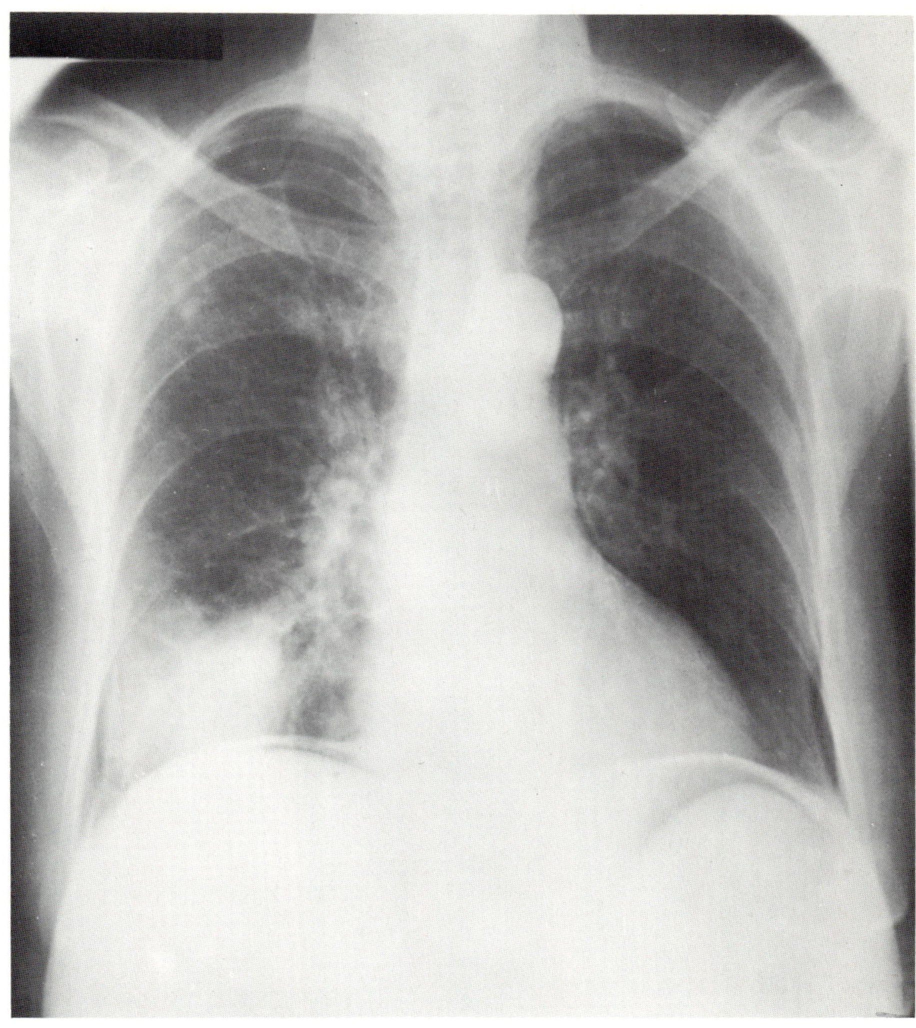

Fig. 42. Right basal pneumonia.

Chapter 3
Genito-urinary System

Calculi in the urinary tract may produce acute abdominal pain by causing renal or ureteric colic or by predisposing to attacks of urinary infection—either pyelonephritis or cystitis.

The majority of urinary calculi are radio-opaque but many of those causing colic are small and thus difficult to see on a plain X-ray. A view of the pelvis with the X-ray tube angled 20–30° caudally should be taken, in addition to the usual plain films of the abdomen and chest, so that small calculi at the lower end of the ureter do not overlie the opacity of the sacrum (see Fig. 50).

In a patient with ureteric colic an increase in quantity of intestinal gas due to secondary paralytic (adynamic) ileus may cause further difficulty in identifying a small calculus. It is in these circumstances that emergency excretory urography is invaluable in reaching a diagnosis. This investigation will also decide whether a small opacity in the region of the ischial spine on the plain X-ray is a phlebolith or a calculus (see Fig. 51). Ultrasonography is not as useful as when identifying gallstones. The soft tissue outlines of the kidney and bladder are due to the enveloping perinephric and extraperitoneal fat. In the patient with abdominal pain abnormalities of these outlines may be of diagnostic value, e.g. ruptured kidney (Fig. 61), perinephric abscess (Figs 48 and 49). As the perinephrenic fat may remain after a nephrectomy a false 'kidney' shadow may rarely cause confusion on a plain X-ray.

Renal calculus (staghorn calculus) Fig. 43

X-RAY APPEARANCES (Supine film)

Staghorn calculus on the left.
Clear outline of the left kidney with preservation of the renal parenchyma.

Other unrelated features

Overlapping outlines and shadows of the right kidney and the liver.
Lower pole of the spleen, arrowed.
Clear psoas shadows.
Thick layer of extra-peritoneal fat ('flank stripe'), arrowed (obese patient).
Lung markings in the posterior costophrenic recess appearing to overlie the upper abdominal viscera.
Rudimentary right 12th rib.

DIFFERENTIAL DIAGNOSIS OF X-RAY

The appearances are characteristic of a staghorn calculus. This plain film must not be mistaken for an excretory urogram, with non function of the other side.

PRESENTATION

Loin or colicky abdominal pain.
Haematuria.
Symptoms of a urinary infection.
Loin tenderness and guarding.

Staghorn calculi tend to occur after prolonged recumbency. In a patient with abdominal pain a staghorn calculus seen on X-ray may only be an incidental finding. Renal calculi should raise the suspicion of hyperparathyroidism especially when they are multiple or recurrent.

CLINICAL DIFFERENTIAL DIAGNOSIS

Hydronephrosis.
Pyelonephritis.
Perinephric abscess.
Gallstone colic.
Prolapsed intervertebral disc.

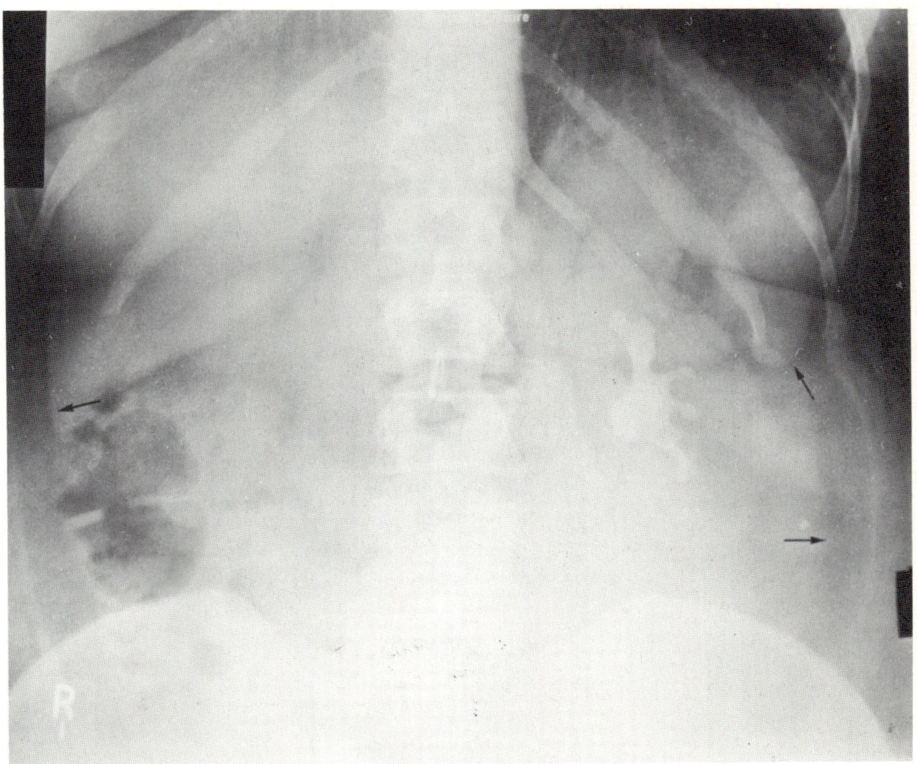

Fig. 43. Renal calculus.

Renal calculi
Fig. 44

X-RAY APPEARANCES

Multiple, bilateral, renal calculi.
The renal outlines are obscured by colonic contents.

DIFFERENTIAL DIAGNOSIS OF X-RAY

Nephrocalcinosis (see Fig. 46).
Pancreatic calcification (see Fig. 14).

PRESENTATION

See legend to Fig. 43.

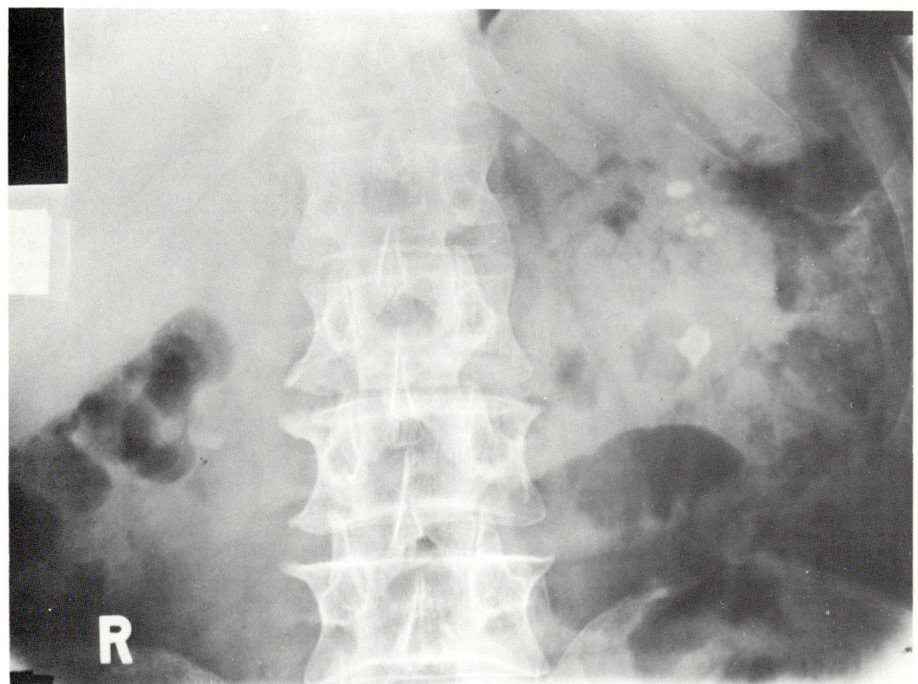

Fig. 44. Renal calculi.

Renal calculus—matrix calculus
Fig. 45

X-RAY APPEARANCES

Large left renal outline enclosing multiple areas of soft mottled calcification.
Normal, although somewhat low, right renal outline.
Prominent (unrelated) calcification of the costal cartilages.

Calcification occurs within the mucoid cast of a dilated pelvicalcyeal system, the cast forming secondarily to an infection usually with Bacillus proteus. The cause of the initial dilatation may be congenital or acquired obstruction, or long standing reflux. Recurrent matrix calculi are not uncommon.

PRESENTATION AND DIFFERENTIAL DIAGNOSIS OF X-RAY

Intractable urinary infection.
See legend to Fig. 43.

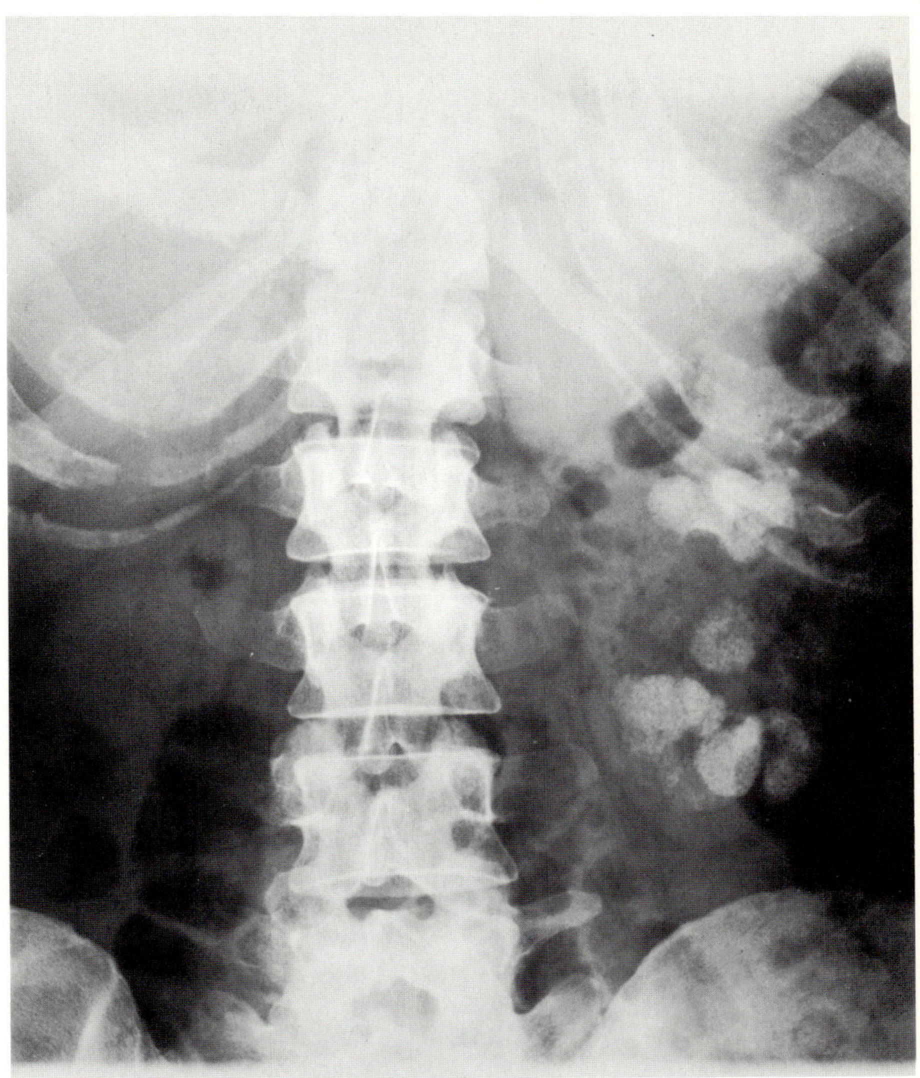

Fig. 45. Renal calculus—matrix calculus.

Renal calcification—medullary sponge kidney Fig. 46

X-RAY APPEARANCES

Aggregations of small calculi 'in the line of' the renal pyramids on both sides. The calculi form in cystic dilatations of the collecting tubules in the renal pyramids.
Obscured right psoas shadow.

DIFFERENTIAL DIAGNOSIS OF X-RAY

Other causes of nephrocalcinosis e.g. hyperparathyroidism, renal tubular acidosis, chronic pyelonephritis.
Renal tuberculosis.
Calcification following renal cortical necrosis.
Chronic pancreatitis.
Calcification in an abdominal aortic aneurysm.
Calcified mesenteric or aortic lymph glands.

PRESENTATION

Ureteric colic. If a cyst in the pyramid ruptures, the calculi are liberated into the renal pelvis and ureter and may either be passed, or retained to provide a nucleus for a larger calculus.
Haematuria.
Uraemia.
An incidental X-ray finding.

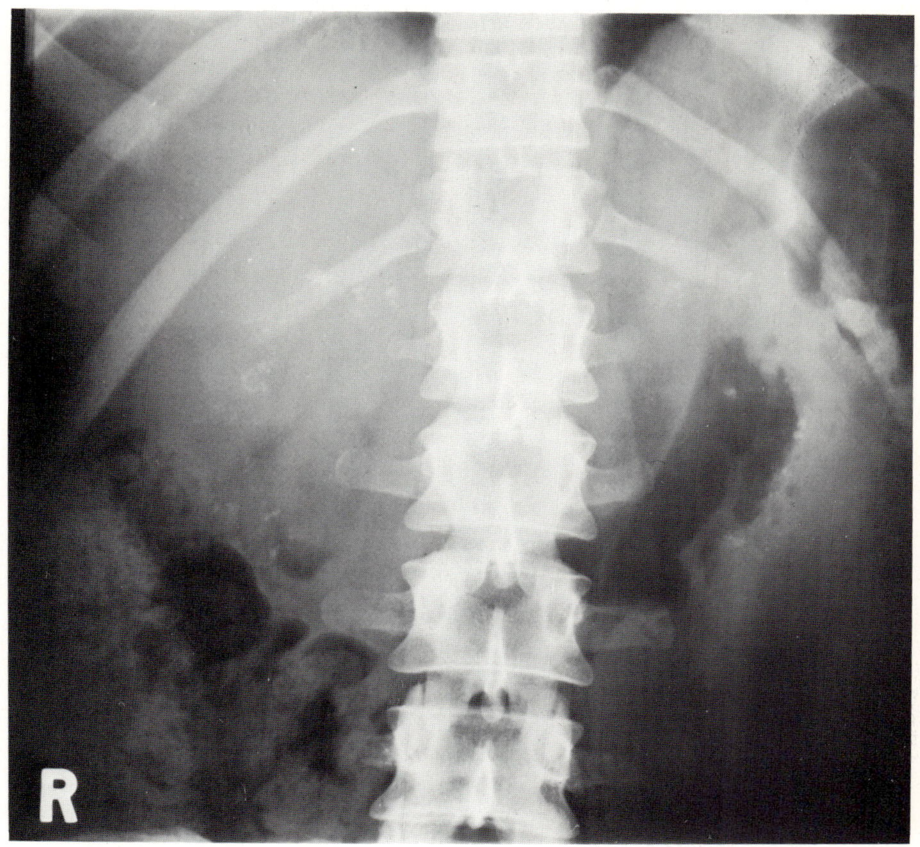

Fig. 46. Renal calcification: medullary sponge kidney.

Renal calcification—calcified pyonephrosis
Fig. 47

X-RAY APPEARANCES

Calcification throughout the substance of the left kidney.
Calcification in the line of the left ureter, arrowed.

DIFFERENTIAL DIAGNOSIS OF X-RAY

Old tuberculous infection of the kidney and ureter.
Calcification in a renal tumour.

PRESENTATION

Abdominal or loin pain.
Symptoms of urinary infection.
Weight loss, night sweats or other symptoms of systemic tuberculous infection.

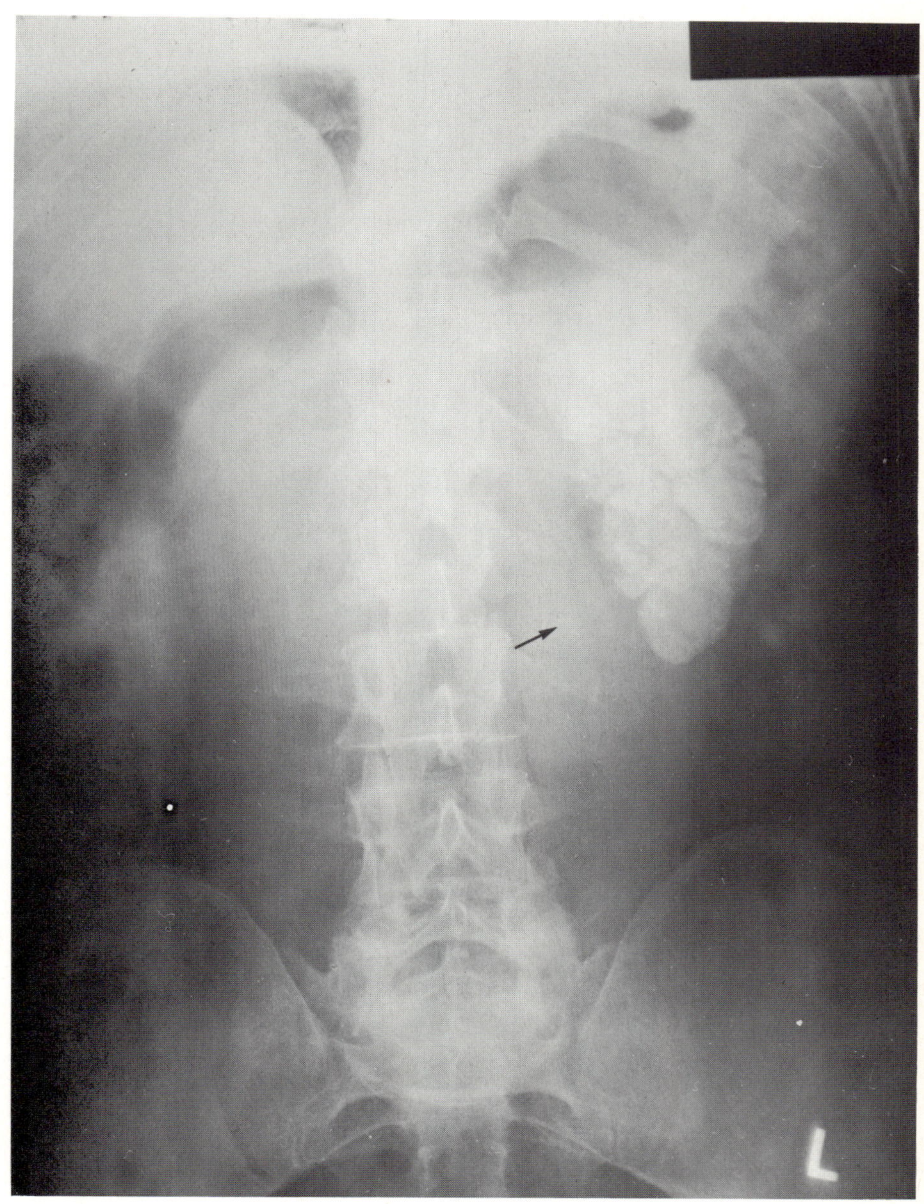

Fig. 47. Renal calcification: calcified pyonephrosis.

Perinephric abscess
Fig. 48

X-RAY APPEARANCES
(Supine film)

Increased width of the left 'renal' shadow, arrowed.
Gas shadows overlying the left renal shadow.
Absence of a left psoas margin due to inflammatory oedema.

The gas has a speckled appearance typical of interstitial gas and is mainly disposed in the shape of an inverted U, being limited by the perirenal fascia. Its appearance is unlike gas contained in bowel, cf. Fig. 24. Retrograde pyelography confirmed the diagnosis of perinephric abscess with gas. The patient was diabetic.

Other unrelated features

Calcified mesenteric lymph glands to the right of L.4 and 5 vertebral bodies.
Ring shadows of gallstones overlying the right 10th intercostal space.
Bilateral calcification of costal cartilages.

Perirenal gas is an uncommon feature of perinephric abscess. The more usual radiological signs are loss of the renal outline or lack of movement of the kidney as seen on inspiration/expiration films or fluoroscopy (screening).

DIFFERENTIAL DIAGNOSIS OF X-RAY

Hydronephrosis.
Traumatic haematoma of the kidney.
Renal or other retroperitoneal tumour.
Distended loop of jejunum.

PRESENTATION

Loin pain with a tender mass.
Symptoms and signs of a systemic infection.
Pyrexia of undetermined origin.
Symptoms of urinary infection.

CLINICAL DIFFERENTIAL DIAGNOSIS

Pyonephrosis.
Subphrenic abscess.
Pericolic abscess.
Degenerating renal or retroperitoneal neoplasm.

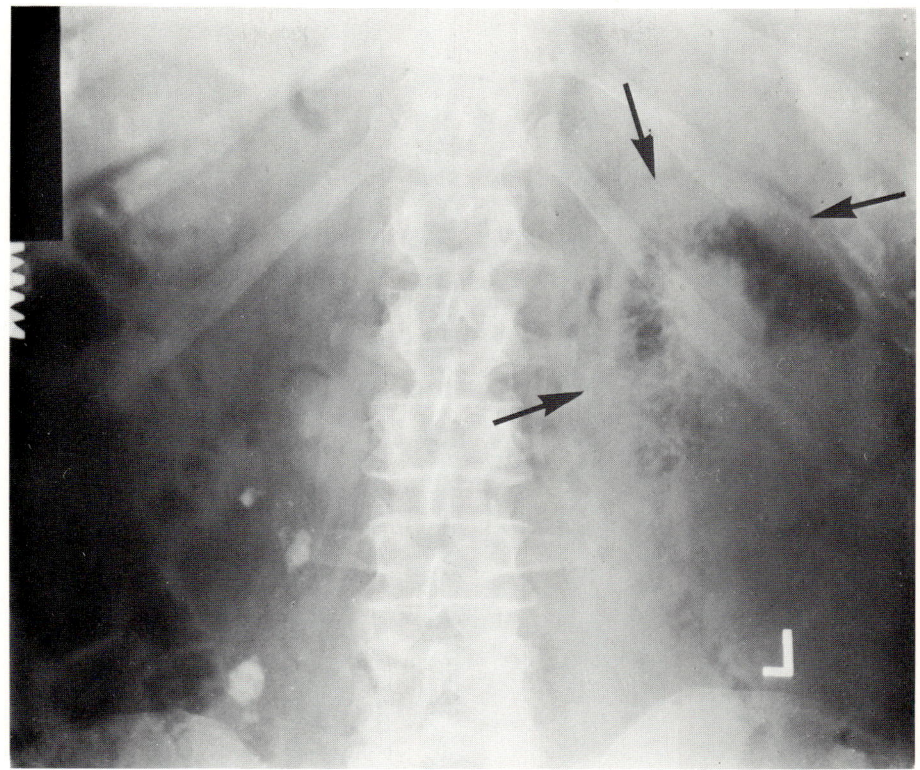

Fig. 48. Perinephric abscess.

Perinephric abscess
Fig. 49

X-RAY APPEARANCES

Well demarcated gas in the right perinephric space, seen better around the lower pole but also outlining the rest of the kidney.

A large stone in the right ureter opposite the transverse process of L.5.

Moderately dilated small intestinal loops centrally in the abdomen.

DIFFERENTIAL DIAGNOSIS OF X-RAY

Emphysematous cholecystitis (see Fig. 15).

Gallstone ileus (see Fig. 18).

Small intestinal obstruction.

Retroperitoneal perforation of a viscus.

Calcified mesenteric node.

PRESENTATION AND CLINICAL DIFFERENTIAL DIAGNOSIS

See legend to Fig. 48.

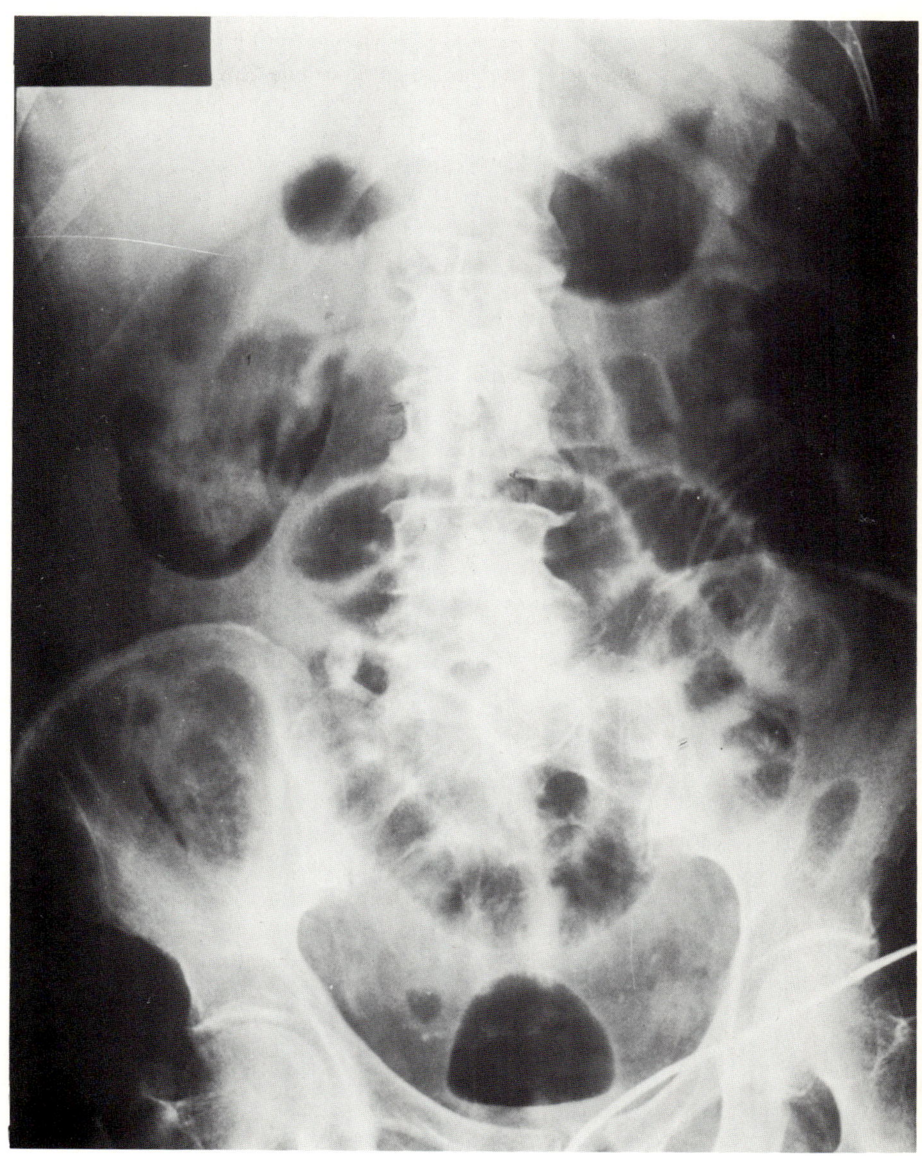

Fig. 49. Perinephric abscess.

Ureteric calculus
Figs 50 and 51

X-RAY APPEARANCES

Fig. 50

Dense oval opacity overlying the right transverse process of the fifth lumbar vertebra.
Two smaller, less dense opacities overlying the right ala of the sacrum, arrowed.

All these opacities are in the line of the right ureter and subsequent excretion urography confirmed them as ureteric calculi. The differential diagnosis of the large opacity from a calcified mesenteric lymph gland may be made by a lateral plain X-ray. An appendicular faecolith may sometimes be seen in the line of the ureter.

Fig. 51

Calculus, arrowed, in the lower portion of the right ureter, at the level of the ischial spine (later proved by urography).

It is unusual for a ureteric calculus to have a central translucency; this is more commonly found in phleboliths (Figs 88 and 90).

Other unrelated features

Symmetrically placed phleboliths in the pelvis. Faecal masses and air in the rectum.
Calcified mesenteric lymph gland overlying the sacral promontory.

The diagnosis of ureteric colic should be confirmed by emergency excretion urography because:
(a) it is important to prevent a diagnostic error
(b) delayed excretion and/or a dilated ureter will suggest obstruction due to a radiolucent calculus
(c) postponement of the investigation may mean the chance of a firm diagnosis is missed
(d) specific treatment, e.g. extradural anaesthesia, should only be instituted when the diagnosis is definite.

PRESENTATION

Colicky pain radiating from the loin to the groin associated with macroscopic or microscopic haematuria, frequency and vomiting. There is frequently a history of previous attacks.
Tenderness and guarding in the renal angle.

When a calculus is impacted in the intramural ureter pain may be referred to the perineum or penis.

CLINICAL DIFFERENTIAL DIAGNOSIS

Acute hydronephrosis.
Renal haemorrhage with colic due to the passage of a blood clot down the ureter.
Acute pyelonephritis.
Acute cystitis.
Acute appendicitis.
Intestinal colic.
Gallstone colic.

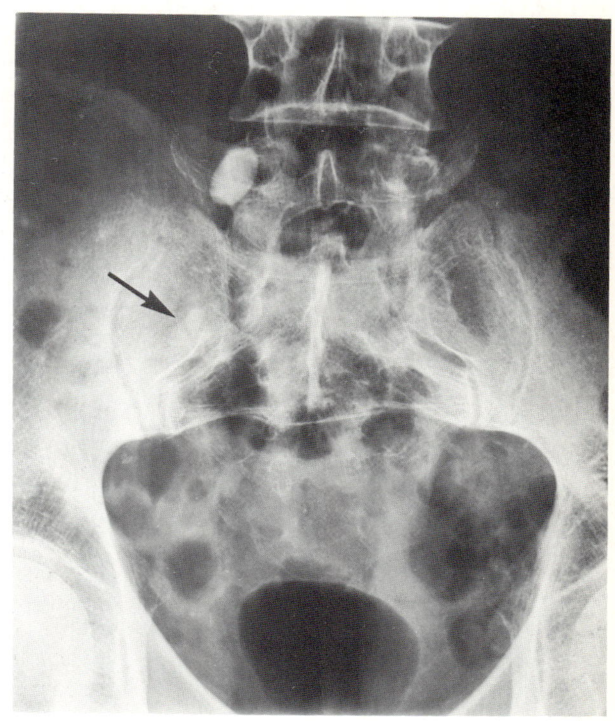

Fig. 50. Ureteric calculus (abdomen).

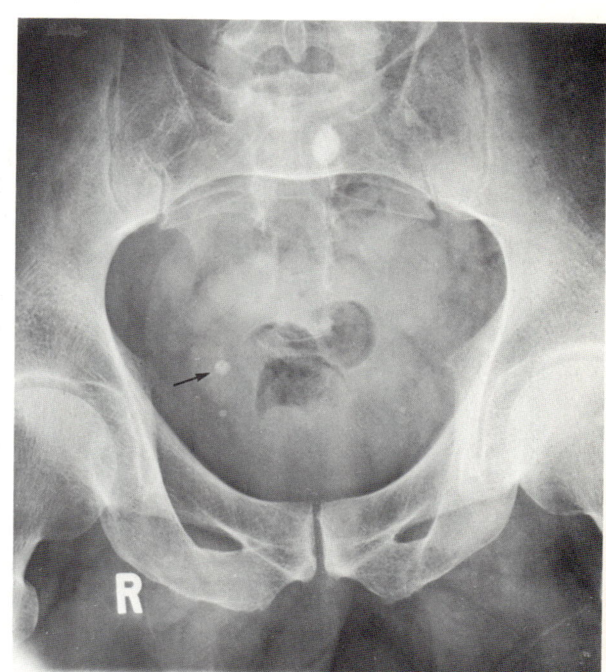

Fig. 51. Ureteric calculus (pelvis).

Vesico-colic fistula
Fig. 52

X-RAY APPEARANCES
(Supine film)

The bladder contains a large amount of gas. Its asymmetry is due to a colonic mass which is seen as a soft tissue shadow in the left of the pelvis.
The rectal gas shadow and faeces are seen through the bladder translucency.

Air in the bladder normally shows an air-fluid level on an erect film. In this instance a supine film only was taken because of the poor general state of the patient.

DIFFERENTIAL DIAGNOSIS OF X-RAY

Gas in the rectum.

PRESENTATION

Pneumaturia.
Symptoms of urinary infection.
Symptoms of sigmoid diverticulitis or carcinoma.

CLINICAL DIFFERENTIAL DIAGNOSIS

Fistula due to:
(a) diverticulitis of the colon;
(b) carcinoma of the colon or bladder;
(c) Crohn's disease of the ileum or colon.
Gas-forming urinary tract infection.
Gas introduced by catheterization or cystoscopy.

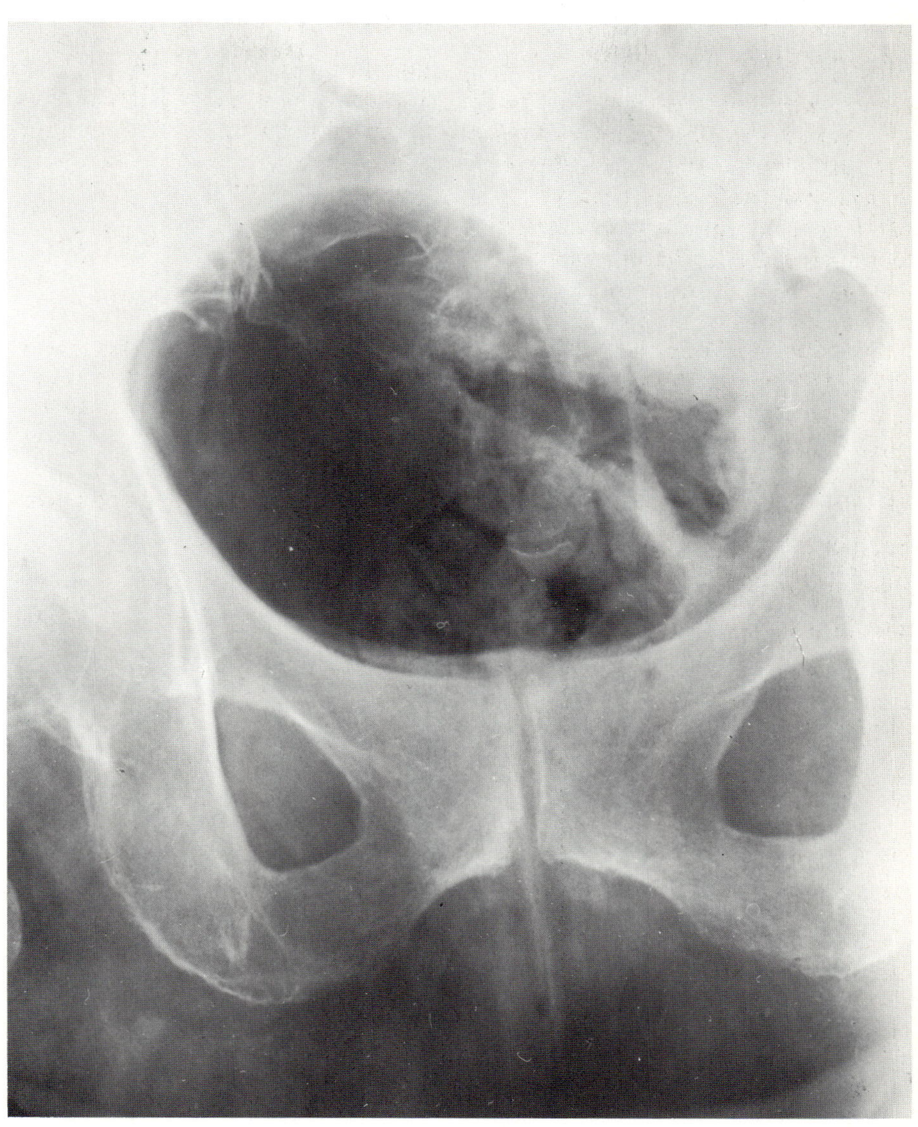

Fig. 52. Vesico-colic fistula.

Bladder calculi
Fig. 53

X-RAY APPEARANCES

Calculi in the bladder, the two largest having a concentric laminated appearance.
Gas and faecal content in the rectum.

The laminated appearance (which is not invariable) distinguishes these bladder calculi from bowel contents or a calcified uterine fibroid (Fig. 89). Calculi may occur in the prostatic cavity following prostatectomy. Fig. 88 demonstrates prostatic calcification.

PRESENTATION

Suprapubic or perineal pain referred to the tip of the penis in the male.
Haematuria.
The symptoms of acute cystitis, often recurrent.
Intermittent interruption of the urinary stream.

CLINICAL DIFFERENTIAL DIAGNOSIS

Acute cystitis.
Carcinoma of the bladder.
Prostatic enlargement.
Prostatitis.

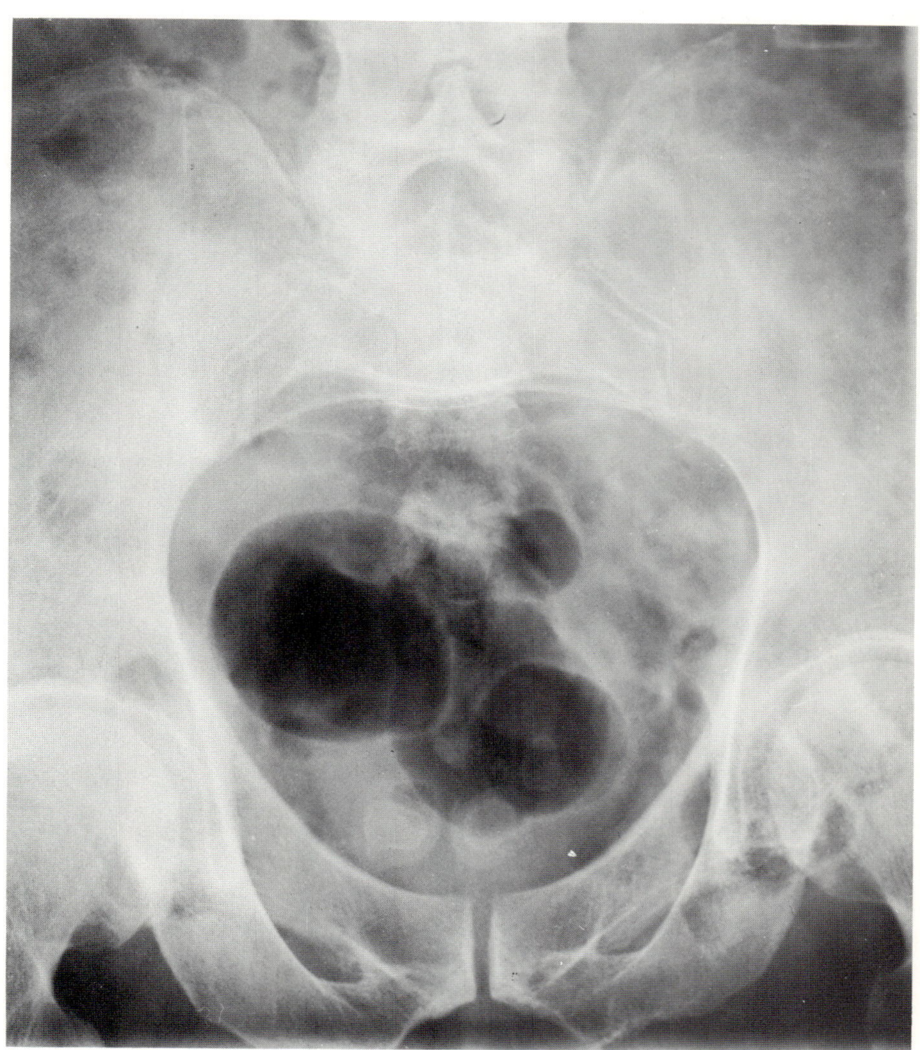

Fig. 53. Bladder calculi.

Ovarian cyst
Fig. 54

X-RAY APPEARANCES

Diffuse shadow in the pelvis, extending into the abdomen. Its upper limit, arrowed, crosses the third intervertebral space and on the right its margin lies within the pelvic brim.

Gas in the rectum and sigmoid colon is visible through the soft tissue shadow in the pelvis.

The remainder of the small and large bowel gas has been displaced peripherally, giving an indication of the size of the mass.

DIFFERENTIAL DIAGNOSIS OF X-RAY

Enlarged bladder.
Pregnancy.
Ascites.
Obesity.

PRESENTATION

Abdominal swelling.

Abdominal pain due to torsion of the cyst or intracystic haemorrhage.

Ovarian cysts usually are bimanually palpable in the pelvis. However, when large they may lie entirely within the abdomen and be freely mobile.

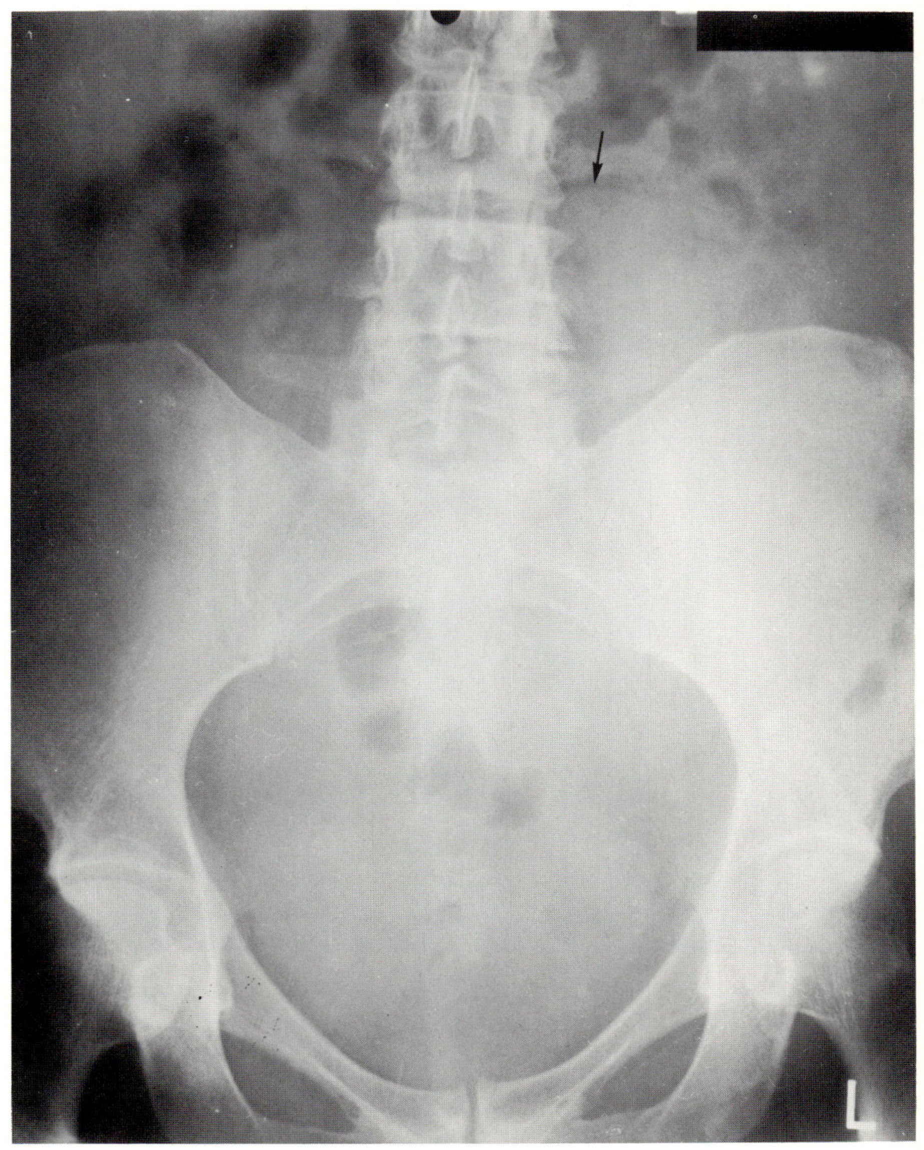

Fig. 54. Ovarian cyst.

Urinary retention
Fig. 56

X-RAY APPEARANCES
(Supine film)

Large ovoid soft tissue shadow arising out of the pelvis. The dome is at the level of the upper border of the fourth lumbar vertebra (approximately the level of the umbilicus).
Intestinal gas and faeces displaced peripherally.

Other unrelated features

Extensive tubular calcification in the iliac and common femoral arteries.
Calcification in both renal areas, probably also arterial.
Osteo-arthritic changes in the lumbar spine.

DIFFERENTIAL DIAGNOSIS OF X-RAY

Ovarian cyst.
Pregnancy.

PRESENTATION

Inability to pass urine associated with acute lower abdominal pain and tenderness.
Incontinence resulting from chronic retention with overflow.
Uraemia.
A cystic abdominal mass arising from the pelvis and palpable bimanually.

CLINICAL DIFFERENTIAL DIAGNOSIS

Ascites.
Obesity.
Ovarian cyst.
Pregnancy.
Renal failure.
Anuria.
Polyuria.

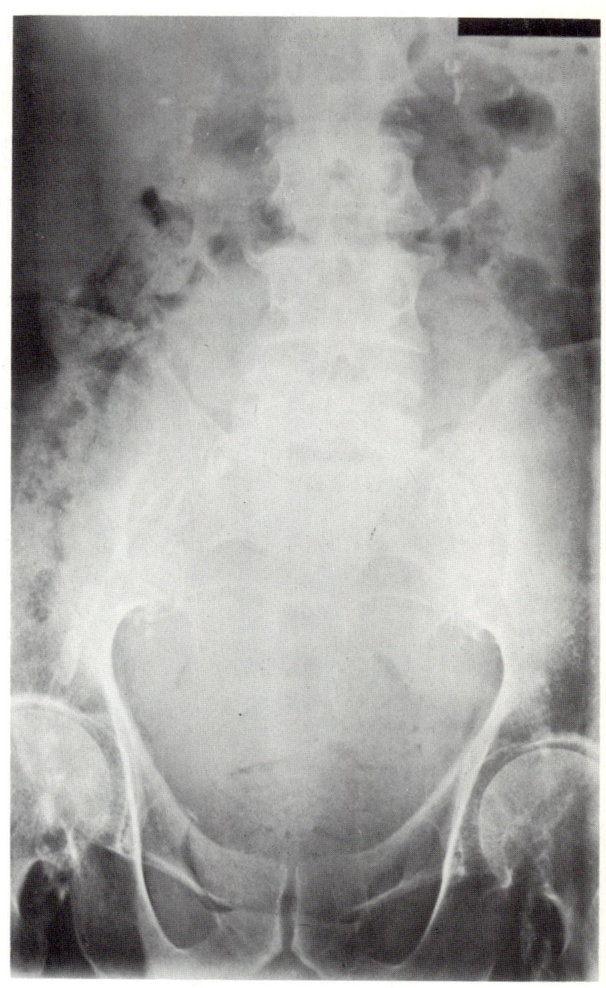

Fig. 56. Urinary retention.

Vaginal tampon
Fig. 57

X-RAY APPEARANCES

The cylindrical translucency is caused by air within the absorbent tampon.

Whilst the X-ray appearances of an intrauterine contraceptive device are well known, those produced by a tampon may cause confusion when the X-ray has been taken to assist in the diagnosis of abdominal pain.

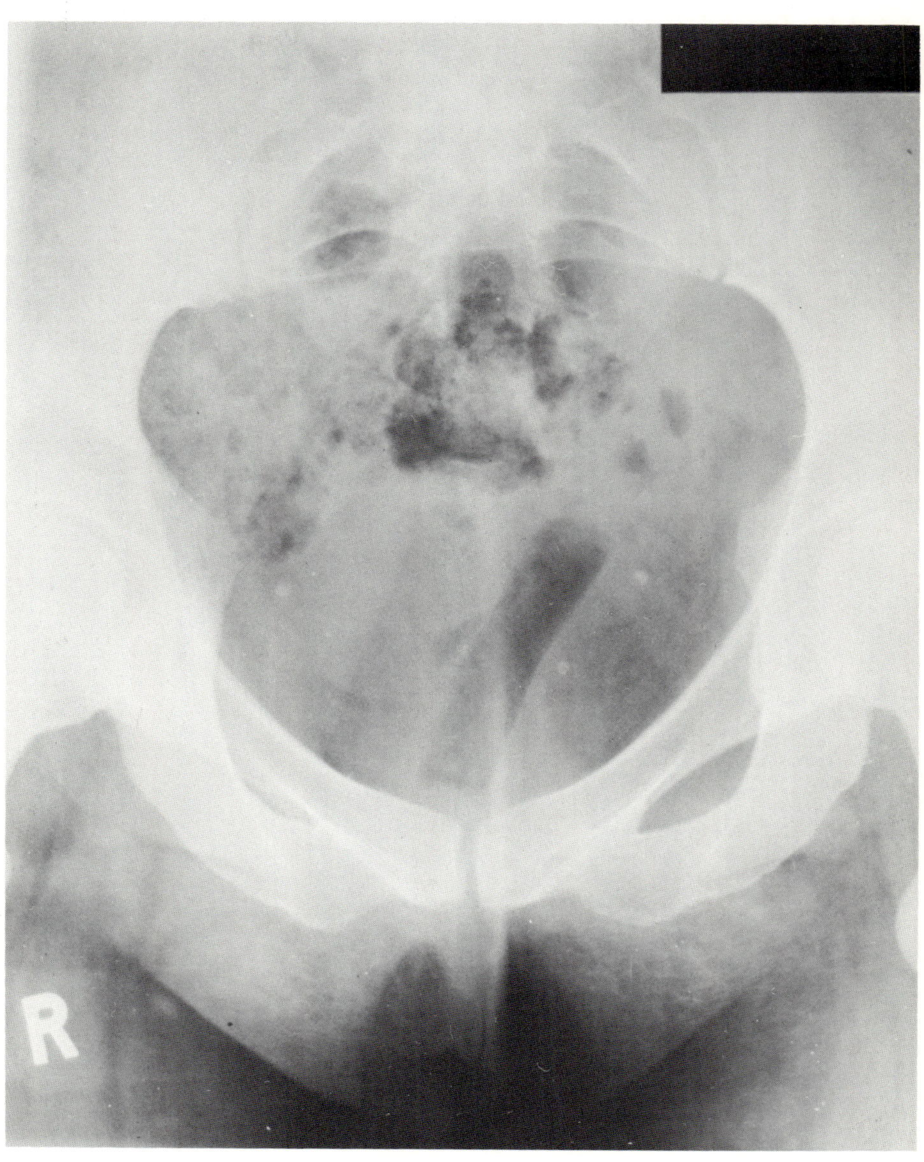

Fig. 57. Vaginal tampon.

Pregnancy
Fig. 58

X-RAY APPEARANCES

A tilted view of the pelvis showing a soft tissue mass within which there is apparently irregular calcification. The tilting is designed to separate this calcification from the sacral shadow. This is the radiograph of a 16 week pregnancy, the woman having requested a termination.

Enquiry regarding the possibility of pregnancy should be made of every woman of child-bearing age before an abdominal X-ray is considered. Radiation should be avoided particularly in the first trimester of pregnancy.

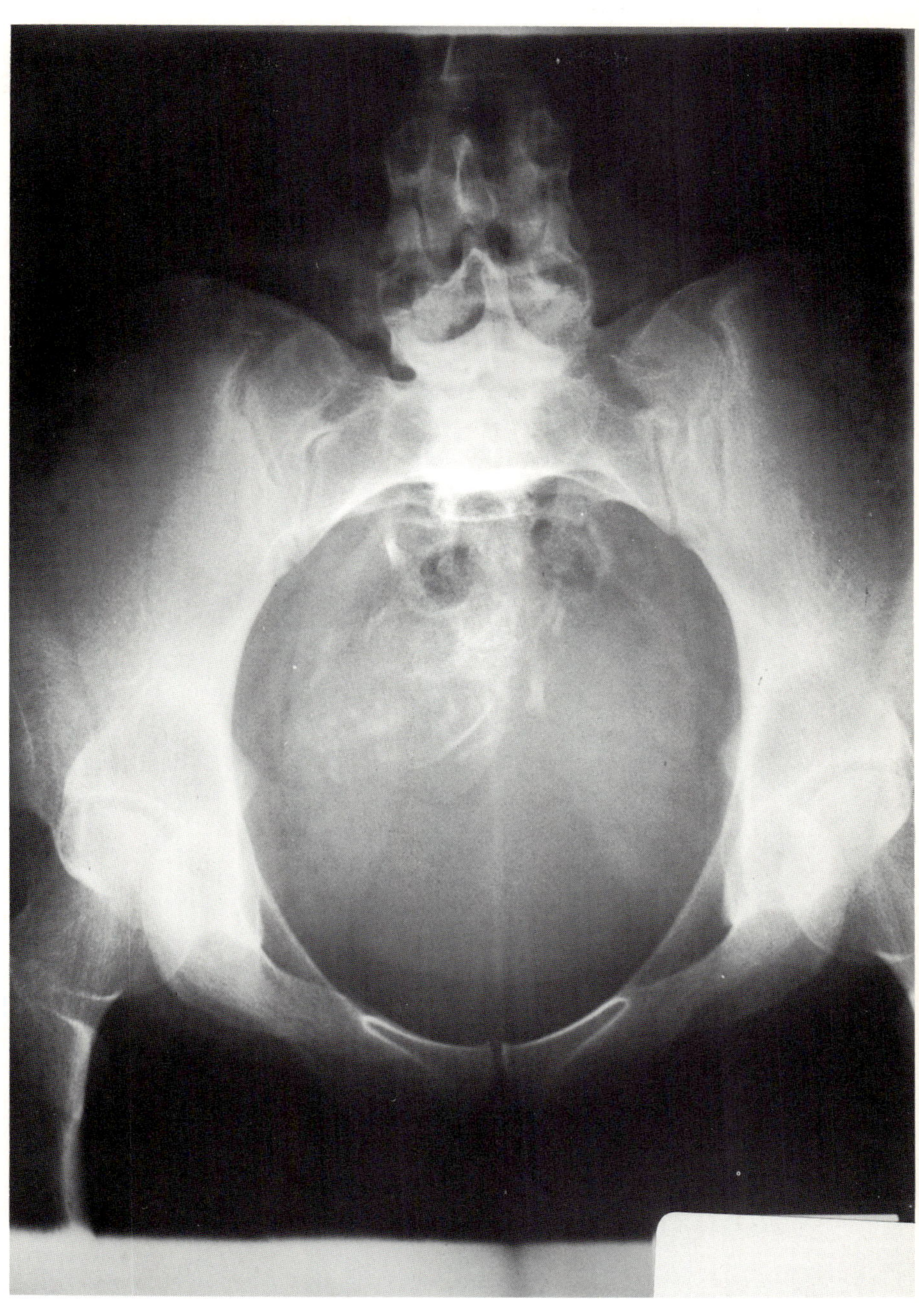

Fig. 58. Pregnancy.

Chapter 4
Trauma

Injuries to the abdomen are caused by penetrating wounds or blunt trauma. A penetrating abdominal wound usually demands surgery, as visceral damage cannot be excluded clinically or radiographically. Blunt trauma to the abdomen is frequently associated with other major injuries and the diagnosis of abdominal symptoms and signs in such patients may be complicated by the effects of head injury, or shock due to blood loss. X-rays are particularly helpful in these circumstances and may conveniently be obtained during the period of resuscitation. As mentioned in the Introduction a trolley with a radiolucent top when used in conjunction with a pedestal Bucky greatly facilitates the radiographer's task, and avoids unnecessary movement of the patient. It also allows the usual abdominal and chest films to be supplemented by films of the pelvis, skull, spine and limbs.

In patients with multiple injuries in whom the clinical picture may be dominated by more obvious lesions multiple X-rays often reveal unsuspected major injuries such as a dislocated hip or a fractured vertebra (see Fig. 64). Such knowledge of the number and sites of fractures helps to assess blood loss. If the degree of shock is out of proportion to the estimated blood loss and intra-abdominal or intrathoracic injury should be suspected. The radiographical signs in patients with the more common visceral injuries are seen in Figs 59 to 62. When the small intestine has been ruptured leakage of its contents produces the clinical picture of peritonitis, and the radiological picture of localized ileus. In this injury gas escapes in such small amounts that it is not commonly seen on X-ray.

Fractures of ribs and lumbar transverse processes
Ruptured spleen
Fig. 59

X-RAY APPEARANCES
(Supine film of left upper quadrant)

Fractures of the necks of the 11th and 12th ribs and mid-portions of the 10th and 11th ribs.
Fractures of the 1st, 2nd and 3rd left lumbar transverse processes.
Normal gastric and colonic gas shadows.
Absent psoas shadow.
Absent splenic shadow.

With this evidence of severe trauma, rupture of the spleen or left kidney (or both) is likely. Fractured ribs are often not seen on a plain X-ray film unless special Bucky views are taken. Rupture of the spleen resulting in a perisplenic haematoma may displace the gastric air bubble medially. Rupture of the spleen or liver resulting in intraperitoneal haemorrhage may produce a diffuse 'ground glass' appearance on the abdominal X-ray. The chest X-ray will help to differentiate right-sided haemothorax from a ruptured liver.

PRESENTATION

History of severe trauma to the left side of the trunk, often in a road traffic accident.
Pain in the left shoulder tip.
Tenderness over the fracture sites.
Signs of intraperitoneal bleeding, viz. abdominal distension; tenderness and rebound tenderness; dullness to percussion and shock out of proportion to the blood loss expected from the bony injuries.

CLINICAL DIFFERENTIAL DIAGNOSIS

Damage to other viscera, e.g. liver, gut.
Haemothorax.
Ruptured diaphragm.

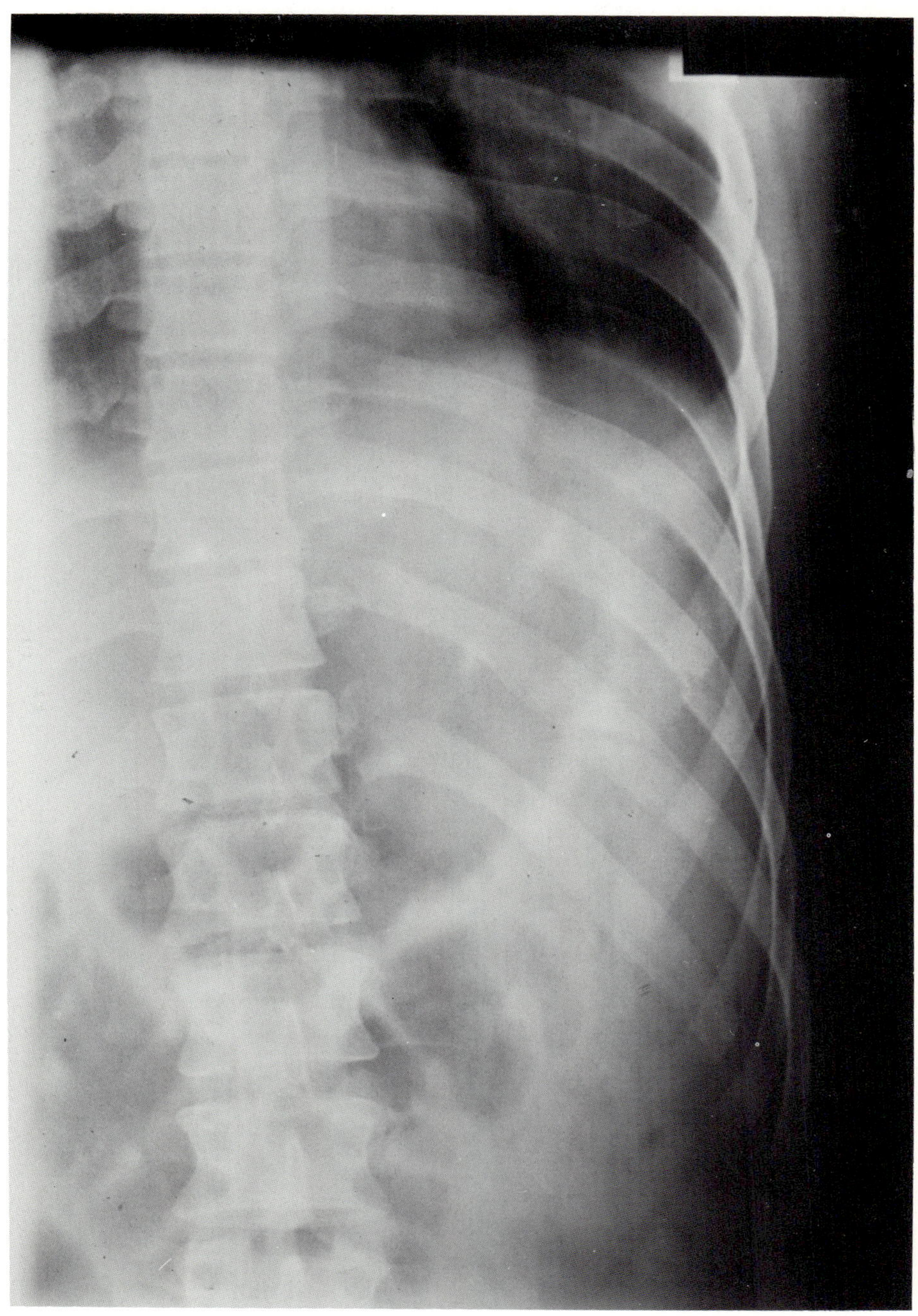

Fig. 59. Fracture of ribs and lumbar transverse processes. Rupture of the spleen.

Ruptured spleen
Fig. 60

X-RAY APPEARANCES
(Supine film)

Gastric dilatation.
Localized paralytic ileus of the splenic flexure of the colon and an adjacent jejunal loop.
Absence of bone injury.

These changes are non-specific but in conjunction with the clinical features suggest the diagnosis of ruptured spleen. The gastric outline is not displaced as this was an intraperitoneal rupture without a large perisplenic haematoma. In the absence of excess air in the stomach, barium may demonstrate displacement of the gastric fundus. Barium examination is particularly valuable if delayed splenic rupture is suspected, and at the same time screening may demonstrate diminished movement of the left side of the diaphragm. Rupture of the spleen may follow only minor injury especially if the spleen is abnormal, e.g. in glandular fever or malaria. The absence of fractures is not uncommon in the young even when there is a history of apparently severe trauma.

PRESENTATION

See legend to Fig. 59.

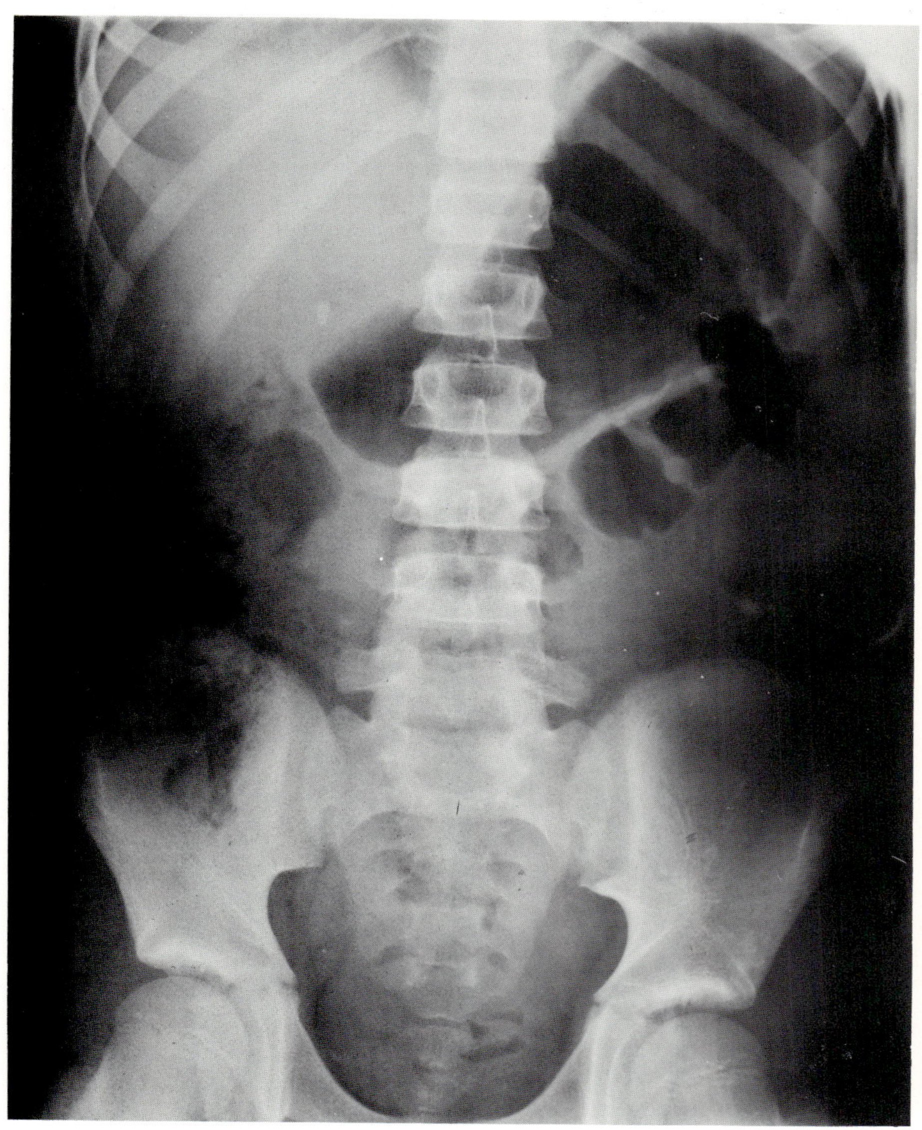

Fig. 60. Rupture of the spleen.

Rupture of the kidney: fracture of ribs Fig. 61

X-RAY APPEARANCES
(Supine film)

Fractures of 10th, 11th and 12th ribs posteriorly on the right.
Lumbar scoliosis convex to the left.
Absent right psoas shadow.
Absent right renal outline.

These appearances suggest rupture of the right kidney with a retroperitoneal haematoma. The scoliosis is caused by reflex spasm of the posterior abdominal wall muscles on the affected side. An excretion urogram should be performed as an emergency procedure. The appearances on the injured side may not be helpful, but it is important to demonstrate the presence of a functioning kidney on the other side.

PRESENTATION

See legend to Fig. 59.
In addition there may be haematuria.

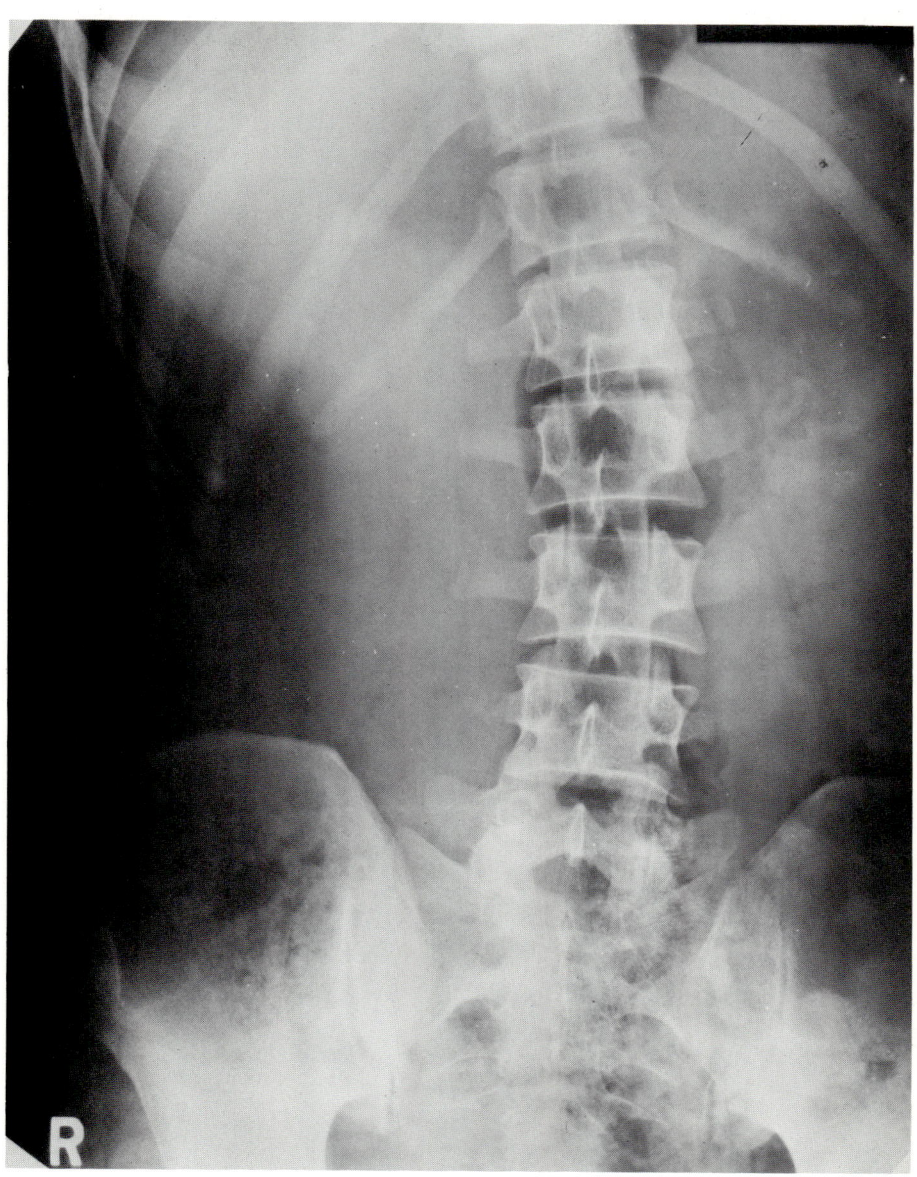

Fig. 61. Rupture of the kidney; fracture of ribs.

Rupture of the diaphragm
Fig. 62

X-RAY APPEARANCES
(Erect chest film)

Marked displacement of the mediastinum and trachea to the right which is evident despite slight rotational distortion (note the position of the sterno-clavicular joints in relation to the spinous process of the 3rd thoracic vertebra).
Absence of the normal left diaphragmatic outline.
Absent normal gastric air bubble.
Distorted gastric air bubble in the left hemithorax.
Gas and faeces in the splenic flexure of the colon, lateral to the gastric air bubble.
Compression of the left lung with resulting increased density of lung markings.

These appearances are typical of a ruptured diaphragm with stomach and colon herniated into the left hemithorax. In the absence of a displaced gastric air bubble the increased opacity above a ruptured diaphragm may be misdiagnosed as basal pneumonia. A lateral chest film should be performed. Owing to the cushioning effect of the liver on the right a sudden rise of intra-abdominal pressure is more likely to lead to rupture of the left side of the diaphragm.

DIFFERENTIAL DIAGNOSIS OF X-RAY

Lung cysts.
Air-containing lung abscess.
Subphrenic abscess.
Haemopneumothorax.

PRESENTATION

The condition should be suspected in any patient who has sustained a crush injury to the trunk, or who has been involved in a high velocity traffic accident.
More obvious injuries may initially obscure the clinical features of a ruptured diaphragm, which may remain undiagnosed for several days.
The diagnosis in an injured patient is suggested by:
Shoulder tip pain.
Respiratory difficulty.
Vomiting, perhaps bloodstained.
Displaced mediastinum.
Basal dullness and diminished air entry.

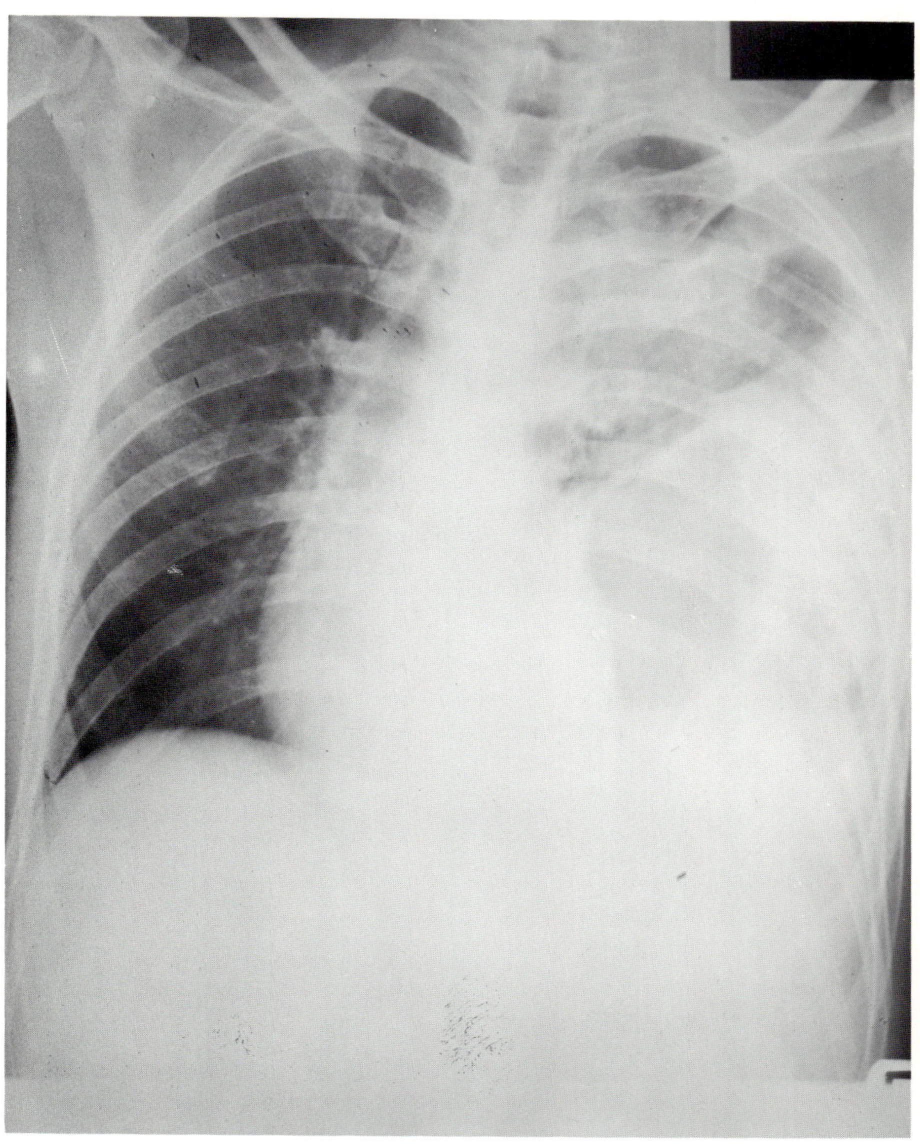

Fig. 62. Rupture of the diaphragm.

Fractured pelvis: fractured sacrum
Fig. 63 (same patient as in Fig. 62)

X-RAY APPEARANCES

Multiple comminuted fractures of the pelvic 'ring'.
Fractures of the superior and inferior left pubic rami.
Central fracture-dislocation of the left hip.
Fracture of the body and right ala of the sacrum.
Diastasis of the symphysis pubis.

PRESENTATION

Severe shock, with pelvic and back pain, in a patient involved in an accident. Blood loss with an injury of this type is usually considerable (see page 119).
The degree of shock and a retroperitoneal extension of the haematoma may simulate intra-abdominal visceral injury.
Associated visceral injuries are common, especially rupture of the urethra or bladder even when the pelvic fracture appears undisplaced.
Injury to the rectum is less common but rectal examination should always be performed.
Complicating nerve or vascular injuries should be sought.

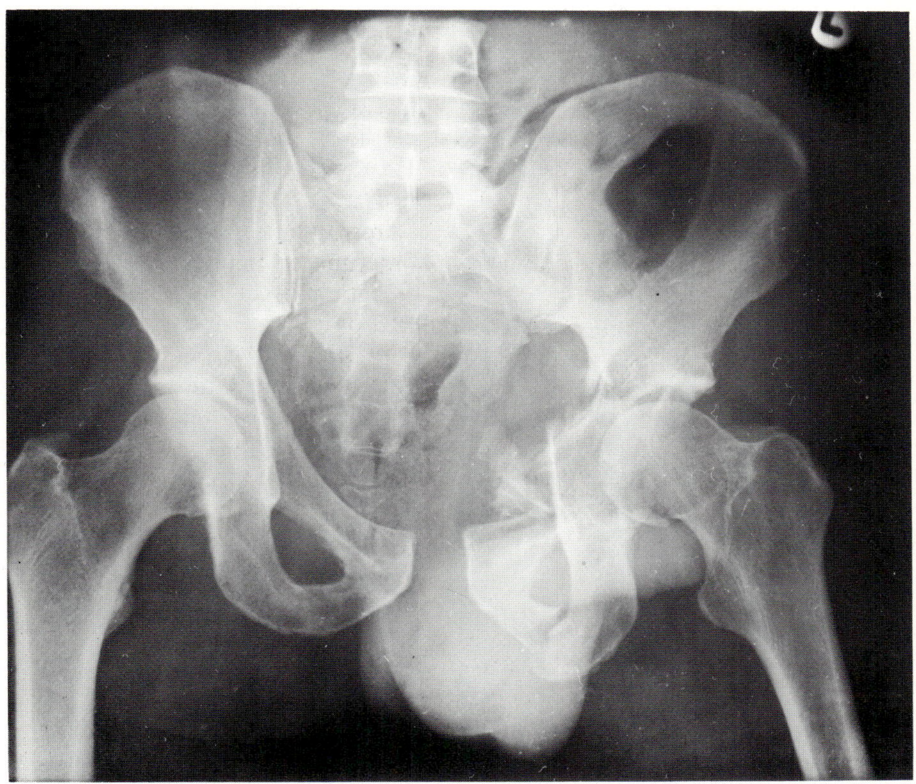

Fig. 63. Fracture of the pelvis and sacrum.

Fracture of a vertebral body
Fig. 64a supine, b lateral

X-RAY APPEARANCES

Supine film, 64a

Lateral angulation of the spine, convex to the left, in the region of the third and fourth lumbar vertebrae.
Lateral wedging of the body of L.4 vertebra.
Diminution of the joint spaces above and below L.4 vertebra.
Incidental spina bifida of the first sacral segment.

Lateral film, 64b

Comminuted fracture of L.4 vertebra with reduction of the adjacent joint spaces. The anterior fragment of the body is displaced forwards.
Despite the comminution there is apparently no intrusion of bony fragments into the vertebral canal, and no associated posterior articular fracture or displacement.

The value of the lateral film in revealing the true nature of the apparently minor changes on the supine film is well demonstrated. The remainder of the spine should be X-rayed because crush fractures may be multiple. Patients with a vertebral fracture giving a history of only minor trauma should be suspected of having bone disease of a generalized or localized nature, e.g. osteoporosis or a metastatic deposit.

PRESENTATION

History of trauma.
Pain in the lumbar region with limitation of movement.
Abdominal pain, either due to nerve root pressure with referred pain or to a retro-peritoneal haematoma.
Sometimes as an unexpected finding in a patient with multiple injuries.
Signs of pressure on the cauda equina, e.g. difficulty with micturition.
Prominence of a lumbar spinous process with tenderness to percussion.

CLINICAL DIFFERENTIAL DIAGNOSIS

Acute prolapse of an intervertebral disc.
Retroperitoneal haemorrhage.
Rupture or dissection of an aortic aneurysm.
Acute pancreatitis.

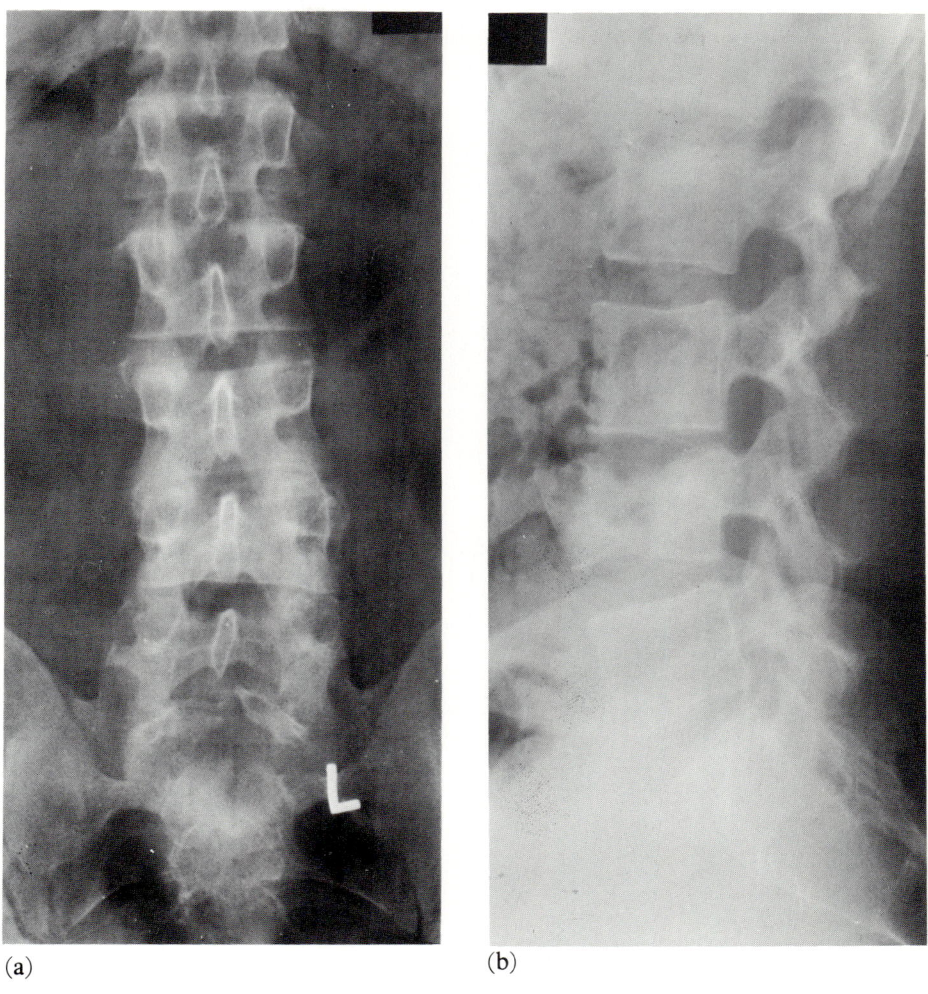

(a) (b)

Fig. 64. Fracture of vertebral body: **a** Supine; **b** Lateral.

Chapter 5
Infancy and Childhood

The diagnosis of the acute abdomen in the child presents a common and frequently difficult problem for the surgeon. The wish to avoid unnecessary surgery while realizing that an operation should be performed early in a patient with acute appendicitis, is the continuing challenge. In the child, as in the adult, X-rays may give helpful information. Acute appendicitis is considered in the child and the adult in Figs 21, 22 and 80. It is in the newborn and the infant with symptoms suggestive of intestinal obstruction, however, that the plain X-ray proves most valuable. Any neonate with bile-stained vomiting should be assumed to be suffering from intestinal obstruction until proved otherwise. A plain X-ray will frequently be diagnostic (see Figs 70, 71 and 72).

The differential contrast provided by swallowed air is usually adequate for diagnosis and it may be helpful to add additional air down a nasogastric tube (see Fig. 70). Radio-opaque media are not often required, should be used with caution, and should later be removed through the nasogastric tube. The inhalation of barium regurgitated from the stomach may lead to respiratory complications and the hyperosmotic effect of contrast media such as gastrografin in the dilated loops of obstructed small bowel in the neonate already depleted of fluids may precipitate circulatory collapse.

Air in the large bowel in infants with Hirschsprung's disease or ileocolic intussusception may also be adequate for diagnosis (see Figs 73, 74 and 78). A barium enema will not only confirm these findings but may be used as a means of reduction of an intussusception (see legend to Fig. 73 and 74).

The frequent co-existence of congenital abnormalities should be remembered both during clinical examination and inspection of the abdominal and chest X-rays of a neonate (see Fig. 67).

In an infant or older child presenting with abdominal pain, lobar pneumonia will be revealed by the chest X-ray, if not on clinical examination (see Fig. 42). Urinary tract infection commonly presents as abdominal pain in the young, sometimes not associated with the usual symptoms of frequency and dysuria. Microscopic examination of the urine is essential in every child with acute abdominal pain. Gallstones, acute cholecystitis, peptic ulceration and acute pancreatitis (usually secondary to mumps or trauma) are all rare causes of acute abdominal pain in childhood. Their clinical and radiological features are described in Figs 5, 13 and 16.

In the very young it is not possible to differentiate small from large bowel when distension is gross because the mucosal patterns are not as well established as in the older patient. Small bowel proximal to a congenital atresia may enlarge to a degree which misleads the inexperienced observer into believing it is large bowel. With less marked distension the air may be more clearly identifiable in large or small bowel, and the contrast it provides may be adequate for diagnosis.

Normal appearances 12 hours after birth Fig. 65

Once the newborn baby starts sucking large quantities of air are swallowed and this may cause gastric and small bowel distension. The radiological appearance must be differentiated from those due to neonatal intestinal obstruction (Figs 71, 72 and 75) or oesophageal atresia with tracheo-oesophageal fistula (see Fig. 67).

X-RAY APPEARANCES

On this film there is a normal distribution of small bowel gas. The descending colon is also well filled and the air has reached the rectum.

The air in the gastric fundus and the small bowel delineates the lower border of the liver, which at this age occupies a larger proportion of the abdominal cavity than in older children or adults.

The opacity overlying the pelvis is an adhesive plastic urine collecting bag.

The soft tissue shadow in the superior mediastinum is produced by the thymus. This is a normal appearance in the newborn.

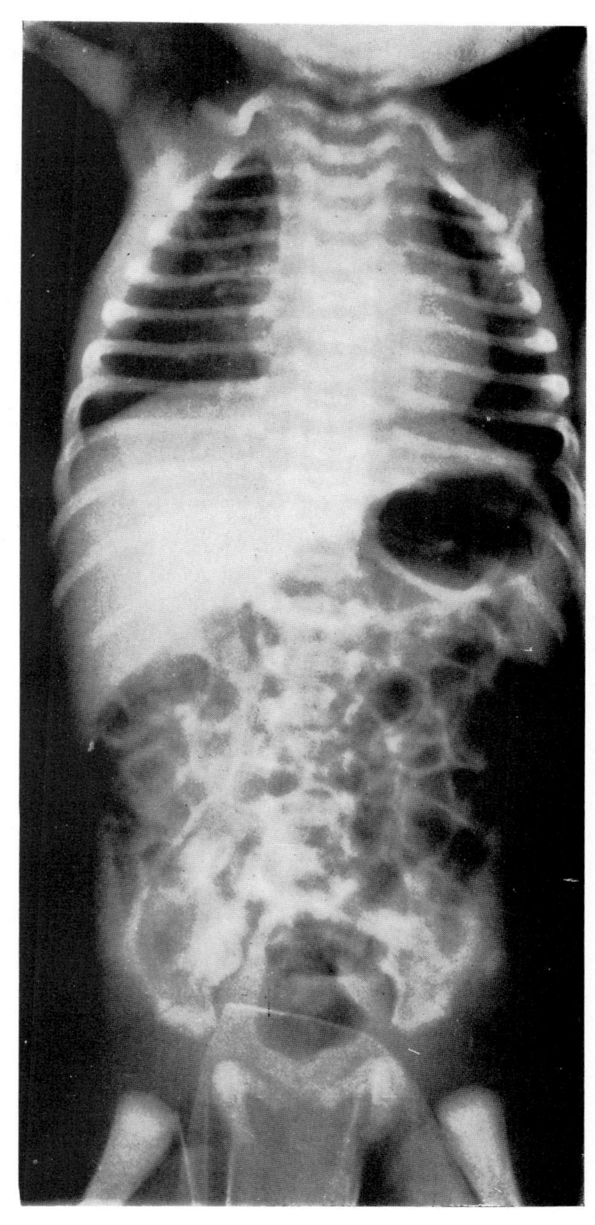

Fig. 65. Normal appearances 12 hours after birth.

Normal appearances in a 9-year-old child
Fig. 66 (supine film)

X-RAY APPEARANCES

Gastric air bubble.

Speckled gas shadows within faeces in the region of the hepatic flexure of the colon. This appearance is common in children, and may extend throughout the colon. Here it is seen also in the sigmoid colon.

Central gas shadow, probably in the transverse colon.

Very little small bowel gas.

Bone island in the right ileum.

Gas shadows in the older child may be similar to those in the adult although there are wide variations in the amount and distribution of gas.

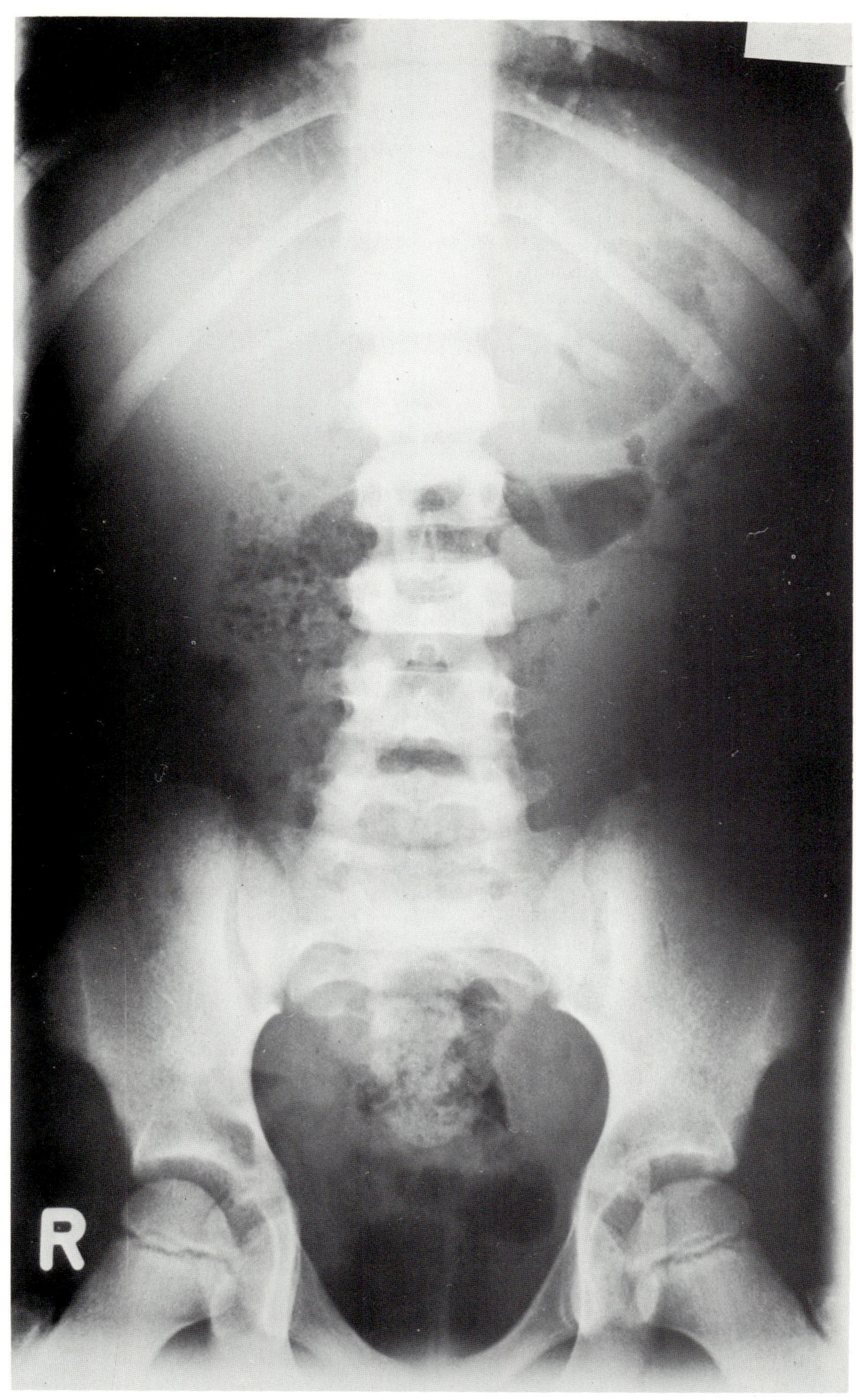

Fig. 66. Normal appearances in a 9-year-old child.

Oesophageal atresia with tracheo-oesophageal fistula Fig. 67

X-RAY APPEARANCES

Stomach and duodenum distended with air.
Some air in the small bowel.
Patchy change at the base of the left lung, suggesting aspiration pneumonia.
Consolidation and collapse of the lower segments of the right lung.
Right pneumothorax.
Bony changes: thirteen ribs; abnormal vertebra at T.5; at least six lumbar vertebra, with fused hemivertebra at L.4.

In the commonest type of oesophageal atresia the lower oesophageal segment has a fistulous communication with the bronchial tree. On crying, air is forced firstly into the stomach, and then on into the rest of the gut, sometimes producing considerable abdominal distension. Unless the other important signs of oesophageal atresia are recognized (see Presentation) a primary abdominal condition may be mis-diagnosed. Aspiration bronchopneumonia results both from reflux of stomach contents through the fistula, and spill-over of saliva or feeds from the upper blind oesophageal pouch. The rare tracheo-oesophageal fistula without atresia usually causes recurrent respiratory infections or choking attacks but may also present with abdominal distension. One major congenital abnormality is commonly accompanied by other anomalies, in this case vertebral.

DIFFERENTIAL DIAGNOSIS OF X-RAY

Duodenal stenosis.
Pneumonia with air swallowing.

PRESENTATION

History of maternal hydramnios.
Excessive frothy saliva requiring repeated aspiration in the newborn period.
Choking and cyanotic attacks on attempted feeding.
Abdominal distension, without vomiting.
Respiratory infection.

Diagnosis is established by trying to pass a naso-gastric tube which arrests usually at T.2 or T.3 level. The passage of a radio-opaque tube makes the use of contrast media unnecessary, unless a fistula without atresia is suspected.

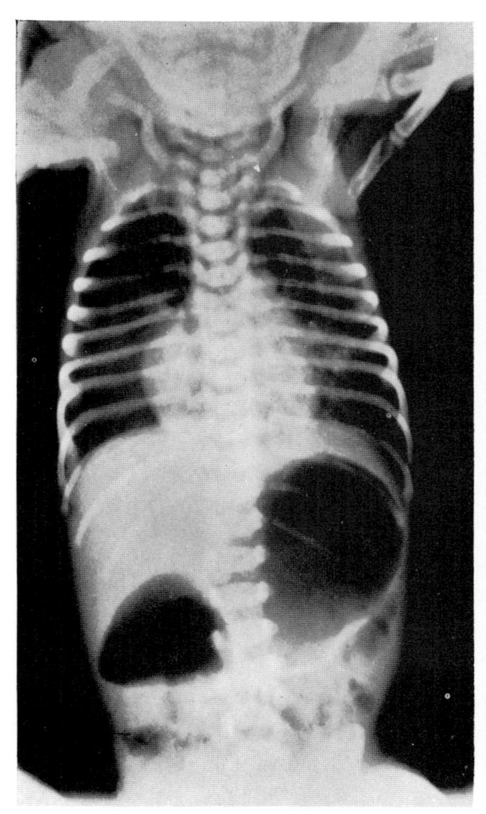

Fig. 67. Oesophageal atresia with fistula.

Oesophageal atresia without tracheo-oesophageal fistula
Fig. 68

X-RAY APPEARANCES

No abdominal gas shadows.

Abnormalities of the vertebral bodies, including hemivertebrae, in the mid thoracic and lumbar vertebrae 1 and 5.

A 'long' baby—thirteen ribs bilaterally.

A radio-opaque nasopharyngeal tube arrested at the level of the proximal oesophageal pouch.

Shadow of the umbilical clip overlying the pelvis.

In this, the long-gap oesophageal atresia, the lower oesophageal segment extends not more than a few centimetres proximal to the diaphragm. Primary anastomosis is rarely possible in the neonatal period.

PRESENTATION

See legend to Fig. 67, but in this situation there is no abdominal distension.

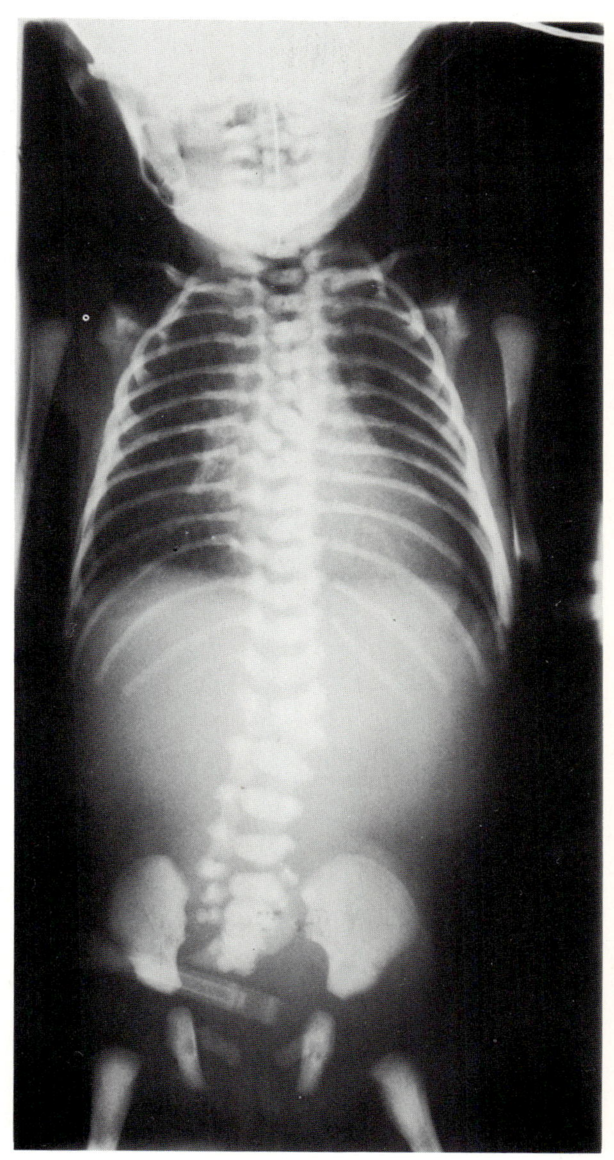

Fig. 68. Oesophageal atresia without fistula.

Congenital hypertrophic pyloric stenosis
Fig. 69

X-RAY APPEARANCES
(Erect film)

Gas-filled stomach fundus with a fluid level.
Enlarged fluid-filled stomach, arrowed, displacing the colon.

DIFFERENTIAL DIAGNOSIS OF X-RAY

Duodenal obstruction (see Fig. 70).

If doubt exists as to the diagnosis, contrast media should be used to study the pyloric region.

PRESENTATION

Possible family history of vomiting in the newborn period, or of proven pyloric stenosis, usually in a male.
Development of projectile, non-bile-stained vomiting between the 2nd and 8th week of life, leading to dehydration and alkalosis.
Constipation.
Visible gastric distension and peristalsis.
Palpable pyloric tumour.

CLINICAL DIFFERENTIAL DIAGNOSIS

Congenital hiatus hernia (common).
Pyloric membrane (rare).
High duodenal obstruction.
Feeding problems.
Urinary infection.

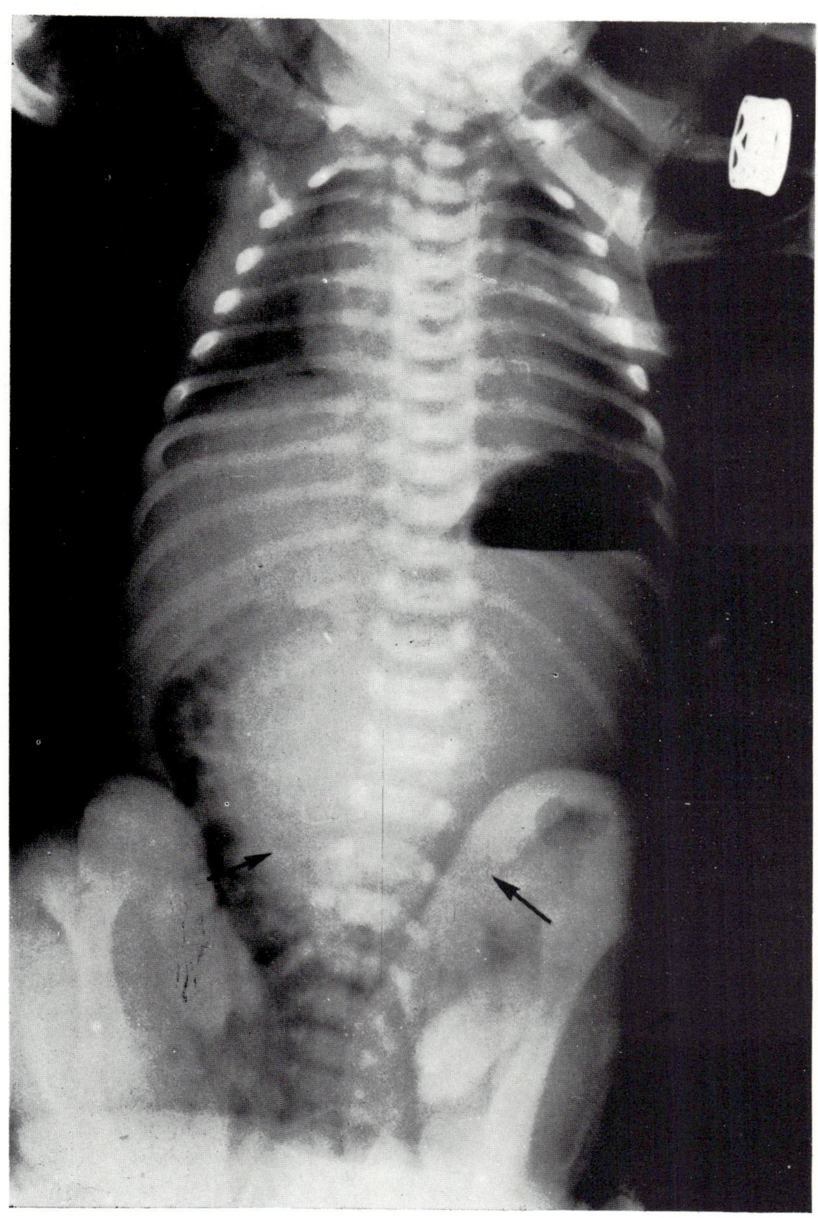

Fig. 69. Pyloric stenosis.

Duodenal atresia
Fig. 70

X-RAY APPEARANCES
(Supine film)

The characteristic 'double bubble' appearance outlining a distended stomach and proximal duodenum.
Absence of intestinal gas distal to the duodenum.
Right pneumothorax.
Unusually dense soft tissue shadow of the penis seen 'end on'.

If nasogastric suction has been instituted when intestinal obstruction was suspected the 'double bubble' may not be marked. Further air may be injected down the tube to provide additional contrast. An erect film will show the appropriate fluid levels. Pneumothorax is not uncommon in the newborn especially when resuscitation with assisted respiration has been required.

DIFFERENTIAL DIAGNOSIS OF X-RAY

The X-ray is diagnostic of duodenal atresia.
Partial duodenal obstruction caused by a perforated membrane, or Ladd's bands accompanying malrotation is not uncommon, but air will usually then be seen in the distal bowel.

PRESENTATION

Bile-stained vomiting, noticed within 24 hours of birth.
Less commonly the obstruction is proximal to the opening of the common bile duct into the duodenum and bile is absent from the vomit.
Epigastric distension.

There may be a history of maternal hydramnios. There is a high incidence of Down's syndrome in infants with duodenal atresia.

CLINICAL DIFFERENTIAL DIAGNOSIS

Annular pancreas.
Malrotation (see Fig. 71).
Pyloric membrane.

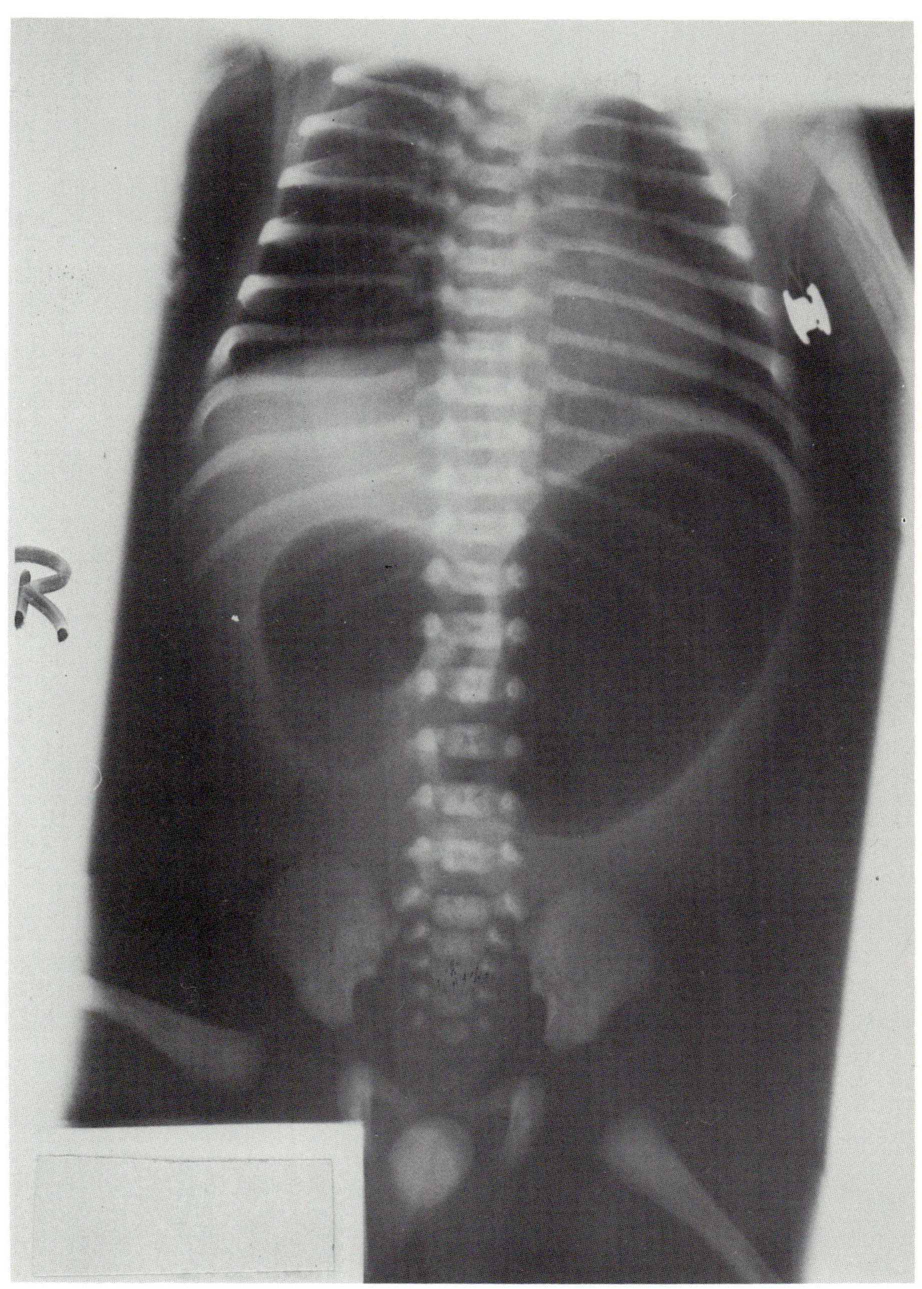

Fig. 70. Duodenal atresia.

Malrotation of the gut Fig. 71

X-RAY APPEARANCES (Supine film)

Stomach and the first part of the duodenum distended with air: the narrower pyloric region overlies the vertebral bodies (arrowed).
Relatively few small bowel gas shadows.
Colonic gas shadows clearly seen.

The X-ray in this condition often does not show specific changes.

DIFFERENTIAL DIAGNOSIS OF X-RAY

Congenital pyloric stenosis.
Duodenal stenosis.

PRESENTATION

Bile-stained vomiting.
Upper abdominal distension.
Failure to pass normal meconium.

Malrotation of the gut frequently presents with these symptoms in the neonatal period. It results from failure of the process of gut rotation and mesenteric fixation which normally occurs during the third month of foetal life. The obstruction is caused either by a volvulus of the mid-gut (which may lead to strangulation) or by peritoneal bands passing across the duodenum from the caecum in its abnormal central abdominal position (Ladd's bands). Malrotation may present in later infancy or childhood with symptoms of recurrent vomiting, failure to thrive, or recurrent abdominal pain.

CLINICAL DIFFERENTIAL DIAGNOSIS

Other causes of neonatal intestinal obstruction.
Gastroenteritis.

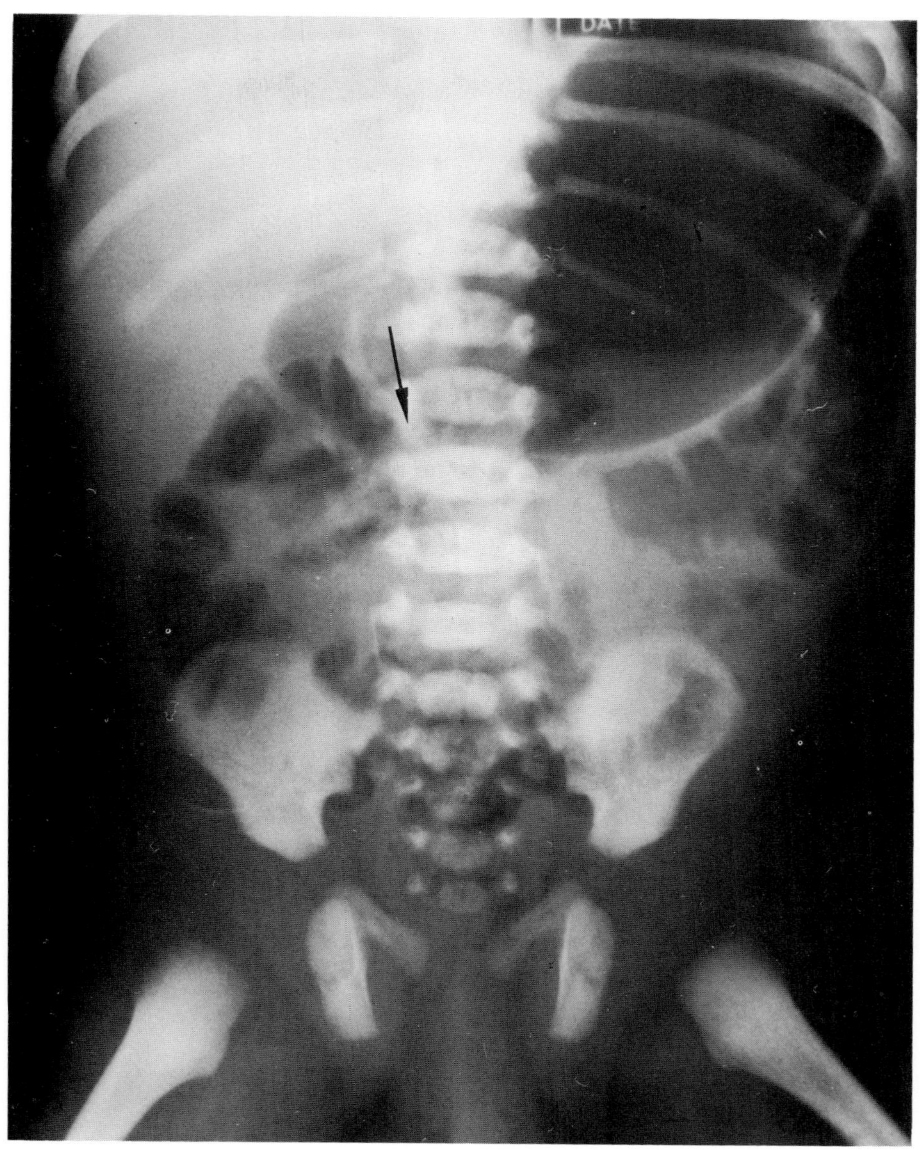

Fig. 71. Malrotation of the gut.

Ileal atresia
Fig. 72

X-RAY APPEARANCES
(Supine film)

Grossly distended loops of bowel.
Some smaller bowel loops visible on the left side of the abdomen.
Normal liver shadow, for a neonate, with overlying temperature probe.

DIFFERENTIAL DIAGNOSIS OF X-RAY

Hirschsprung's disease.

PRESENTATION

Bile-stained vomiting.
Abdominal distension.
Failure to pass normal meconium.

Atresia of the small gut may be caused by segmental mesenteric vascular occlusion in the fetus. The infarcted gut leaks meconium which may later become calcified. As the meconium is sterile healing of the adjacent viable gut occurs. The proximal bowel then distends. If a small vessel has been occluded there may only be an intraluminal membrane causing obstruction: occlusion of a larger vessel or strangulation of a loop results in a wedge shaped mesenteric defect with absence of a variable length of bowel.

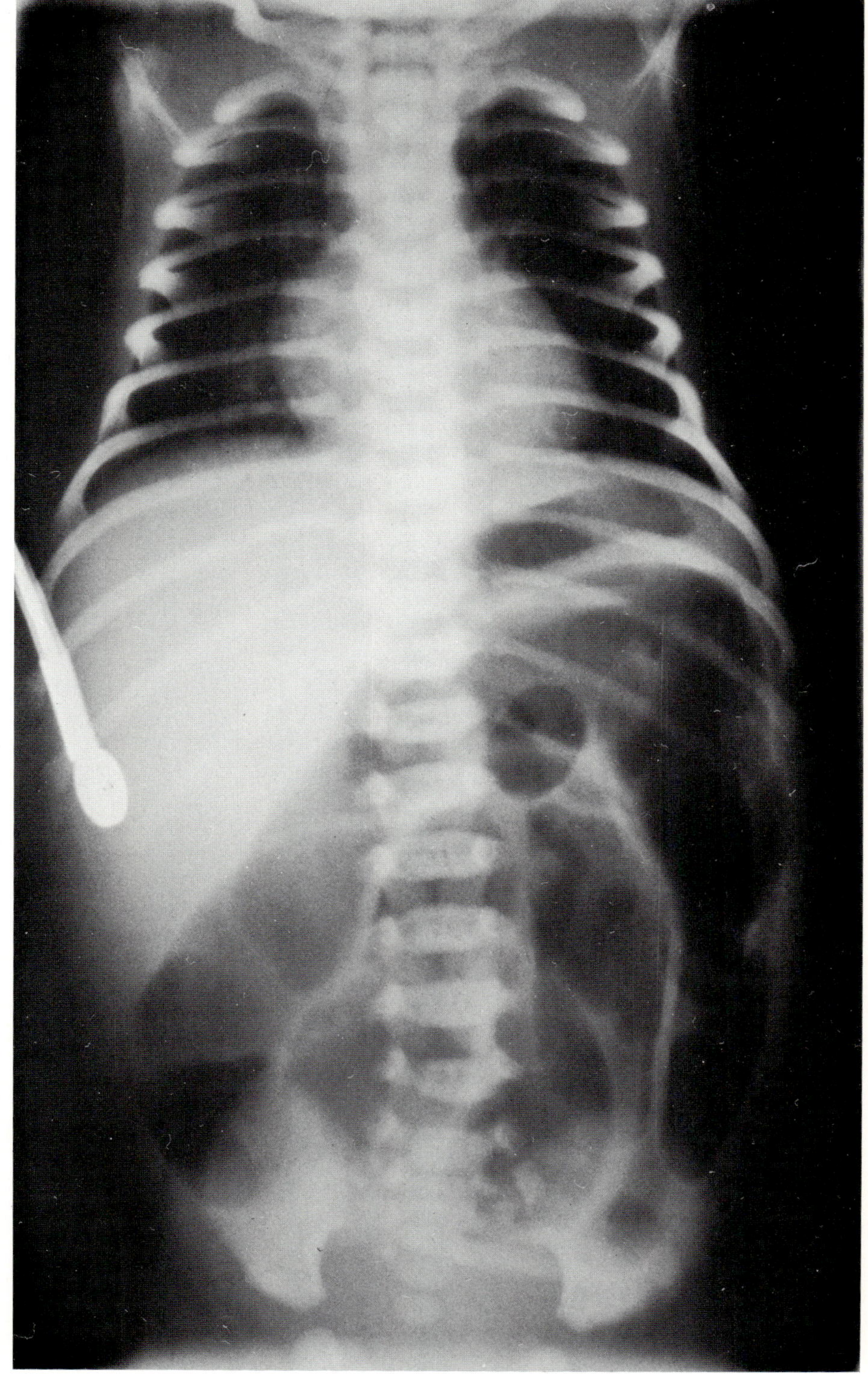

Intussusception
Figs 73 and 74

X-RAY APPEARANCES

Fig. 73 (Supine film)

'Ladder-pattern' of obliquely placed loops of distended ileum.
Granularity of retained intestinal contents.
Ill-defined soft tissue shadow to the right of L.2 and L.3 vertebral bodies, superimposed on the ladder pattern.

Other unrelated features

Normal flank stripe, arrowed.
Bladder shadow in the pelvis.

Fig. 74 (Supine film)

Gas-filled transverse colon.
'Cervix-shaped' soft tissue shadow projecting into the lumen of the right half of the transverse colon, arrowed. This is the apex of the intussusception.
Moderate dilatation of the proximal small bowel.
Gas in the descending colon.

In both these children a sausage-shaped mass was felt in the right hypochondrium. The diagnosis was confirmed by barium enema and the intussusception was reduced under fluoroscopic control by the hydrostatic pressure of the barium.

DIFFERENTIAL DIAGNOSIS OF X-RAY

Appendix abscess with obstruction (cf. Fig. 80).

PRESENTATION

A child of between two months and five years of age.
Episodic acute colicky abdominal pain, with pallor.
Vomiting.
Palpable abdominal mass.
Passage of blood-stained mucus per rectum (red currant jelly stool).

CLINICAL DIFFERENTIAL DIAGNOSIS

Gastroenteritis.
Appendicitis.
Other mechanical causes of intestinal obstruction.
Henoch-Schonlein purpura.
Lead poisoning.

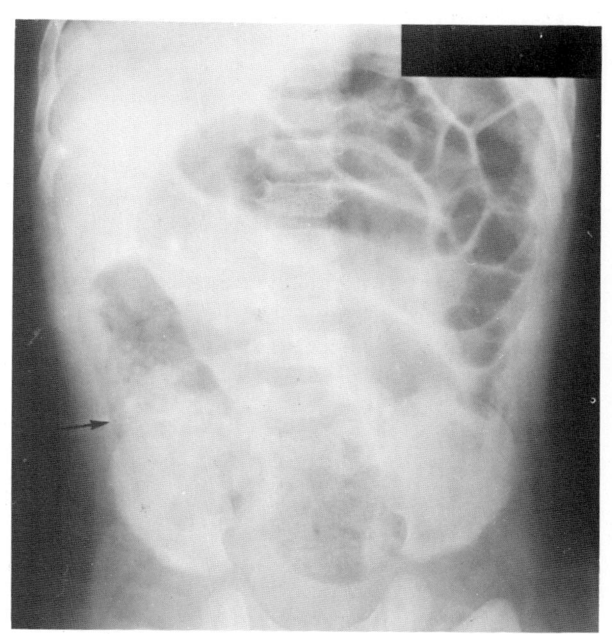

Fig. 73. Intussusception.

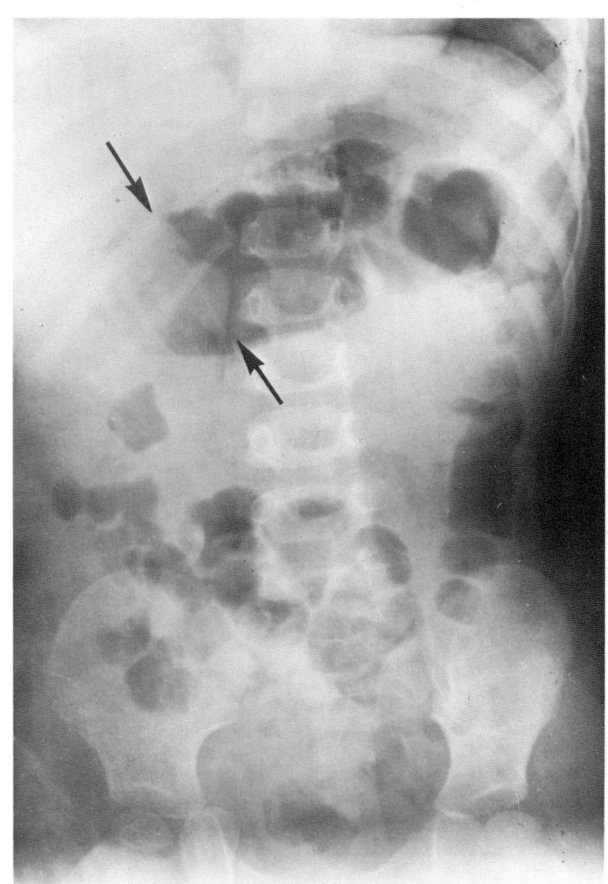

Fig. 74. Intussusception.

Meconium ileus (fibrocystic disease; mucoviscidosis) Fig. 75

X-RAY APPEARANCES (Supine film)

Abdominal distension.
Granular opacity, with included small air bubbles, occupying the right abdomen.
Distended small bowel loops of varying size.

The granularity is caused by inspissated meconium impacted in the distal small bowel. In the mid-ileum it also causes variable degrees of segmental obstruction, hence the differing sizes of the loops. The chest X-ray in this infant was normal but in some patients the respiratory complications of fibrocystic disease (mucoviscidosis) ensue.

DIFFERENTIAL DIAGNOSIS OF X-RAY

This X-ray appearance is characteristic. The granular appearance is sometimes less obvious and Hirschsprung's disease may be suspected.

PRESENTATION

Possible family history of fibrocystic disease.
Abdominal distension.
Bile-stained vomiting.
Failure to pass normal meconium.
Palpable loops of small bowel.
Peritonitis due to perforation.

CLINICAL DIFFERENTIAL DIAGNOSIS

See legend to Fig. 78.

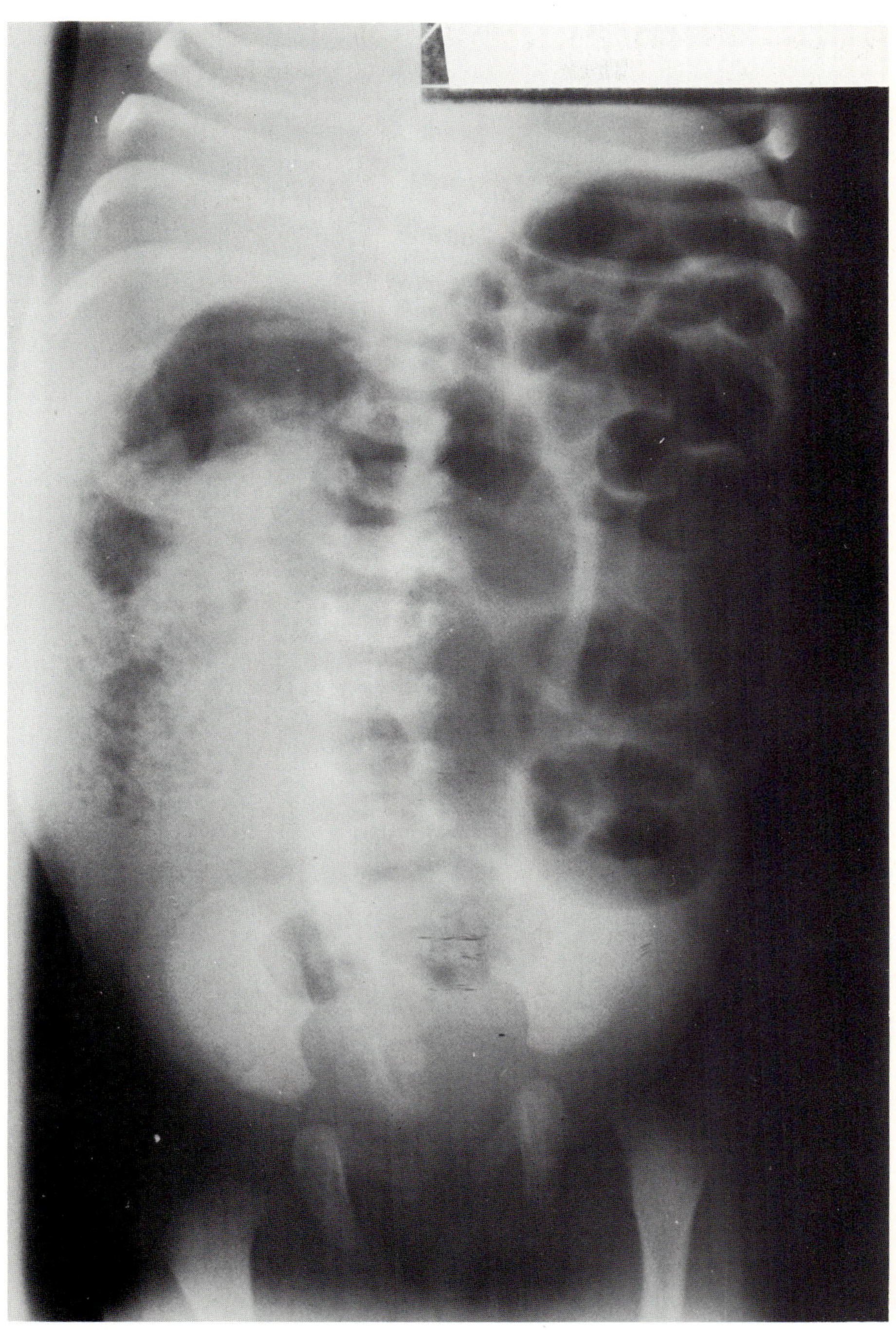

Fig. 75. Meconium ileus.

Meconium peritonitis
Fig. 76

X-RAY APPEARANCES
(Erect film)

Distended abdomen with bowel loops of varying sizes.
Apparently thickened wall of some bowel loops. This appearance is due to mural oedema and fibrin between the loops of bowel.
Widespread peritoneal calcification, most clearly seen in the right and left subphrenic areas.
Thickened abdominal wall on the right. This was due to oedema.
The artefact shadows are of an umbilical clip and a temperature probe.
Normal rectal gas shadow.

This infant had had a prenatal ileal perforation secondary to the intraluminal pressure of inspissated meconium some weeks before birth. The diagnosis of fibrocystic disease was later confirmed. Meconium spilled from the perforation, spread with a peritoneal exudate throughout the abdominal cavity and later calcified. In the male such spillage may sometimes extend through the patent processus vaginalis so that later calcification of the tunica vaginalis around the testes is seen. Meconium spillage may also follow a mesenteric vascular accident which presents at birth as ileal or jejunal atresia (Fig. 72).

DIFFERENTIAL DIAGNOSIS OF X-RAY

Meconium peritonitis secondary to ileal or jejunal atresia, or volvulus.

PRESENTATION

Bile stained vomiting.
Abdominal distension.
Oedema or erythema of the abdominal wall.
Failure to pass normal meconium.

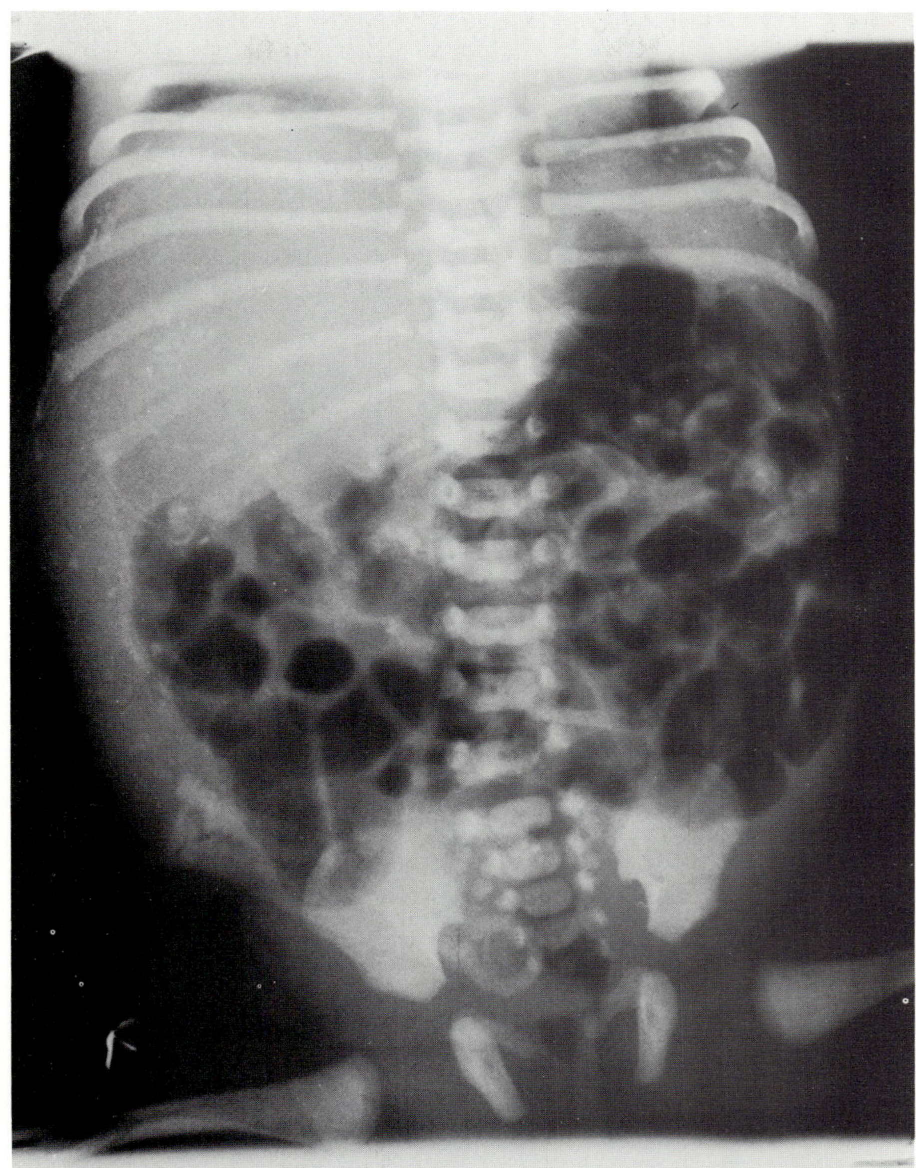

Fig. 76. Meconium peritonitis.

Mechanical obstruction due to hernia
Fig. 77

X-RAY APPEARANCES
(Supine film)

Small bowel distension.
One distended loop outside the abdominal cavity, in the upper scrotum. This is an obstructed inguinal hernia containing bowel.

DIFFERENTIAL DIAGNOSIS OF X-RAY

Once the loop of bowel is recognised to be outside the abdomen the cause of the intestinal obstruction is clear.

PRESENTATION

Abdominal distension, pain and vomiting.
Palpable lump in the groin. In the small boy with plentiful suprapubic fat it is possible to overlook a small hernia.

CLINICAL DIFFERENTIAL DIAGNOSIS

Torsion of the testis.
Hydrocoele with coincident abdominal pain.
Intussusception.
Appendicitis with ileus.
Volvulus.
Hirschsprung's disease.
Band obstruction.

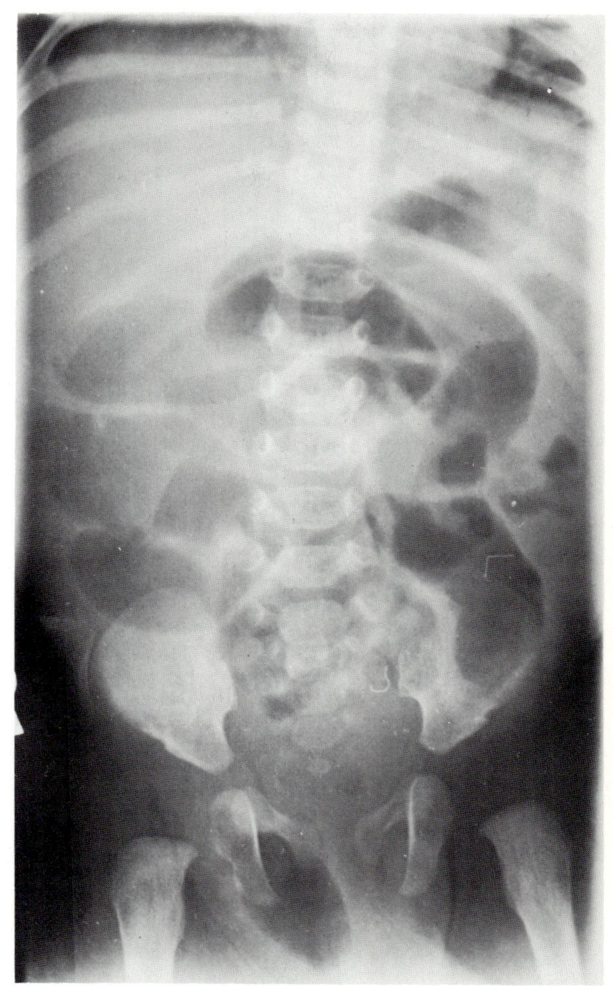

Fig. 77. Mechanical obstruction due to hernia.

Hirschsprung's disease
Fig. 78a and b

X-RAY APPEARANCES
(Supine and lateral films)

Supine film, a

Generalized distension of the large bowel, apart from the relatively normal rectum and distal sigmoid.

Distended small bowel loops. In this example the small and large bowel loops are more readily identifiable than is often the case.

Flank stripe visible on the left.

Lateral film, b

The termination of the gas shadow of the large bowel is cone shaped.

DIFFERENTIAL DIAGNOSIS OF X-RAY

Ileal atresia.

Meconium plug syndrome.

Imperforate anus.

PRESENTATION

Neonatal

As intestinal obstruction, with bile-stained vomiting, distension and failure to pass meconium.

In infancy

As failure to thrive with abdominal distension, often of marked degree, and constipation.

If secondary enterocolitis occurs the presentation will be the same as that of infective gastroenteritis.

In childhood

Chronic constipation.

Abdominal distension.

Often growth retardation.

CLINICAL DIFFERENTIAL DIAGNOSIS

Neonatal

'Meconium plug' syndrome (which occurs usually in premature infants).

Meconium ileus.

Malrotation.

Anorectal abnormality. Except for the rare examples of anorectal membrane or rectal atresia there will be an obvious anal abnormality.

Infancy and childhood

Gastroenteritis.

Chronic constipation (acquired megacolon).

Abdominal mass, e.g. hydronephrosis or tumour.

(a)

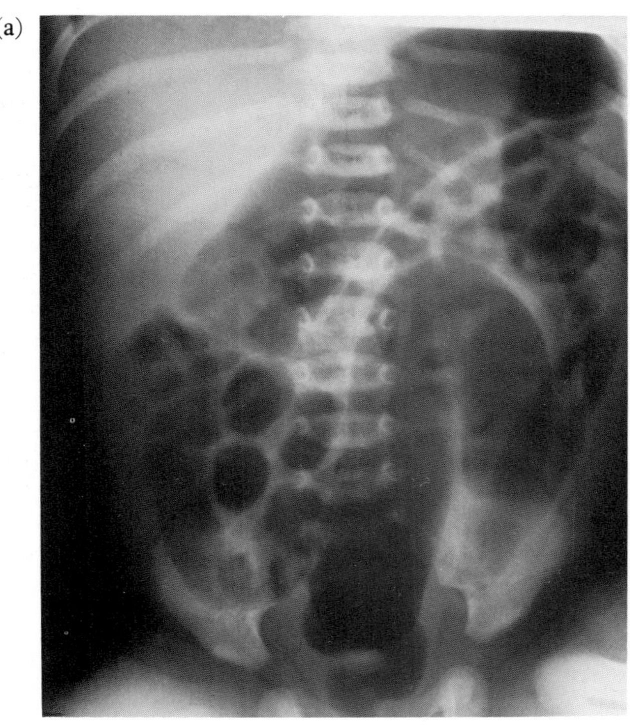

(b)

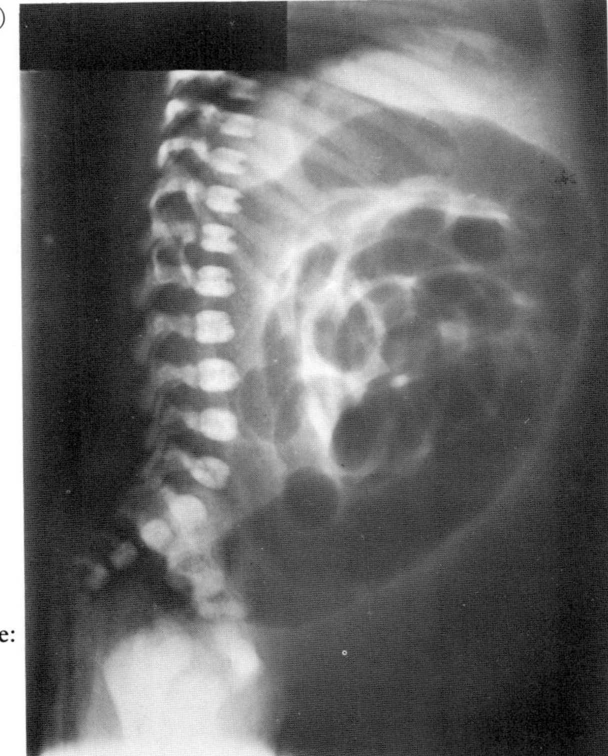

Fig. 78. Hirschsprung's disease: **a** Supine; **b** Lateral.

Necrotizing enterocolitis
Fig. 79

X-RAY APPEARANCES
(Supine film)

Distended abdomen in a small (1.3 kg) baby.

Unusual gas shadows due to dilated loops of bowel, some of which have walls thickened by oedema whilst others show intramural gas.

Thickened lateral abdominal wall, due to oedema.

Pneumonic changes in the right lung.

Radio-opaque nasogastric tube and ECG leads.

Neonatal necrotizing enterocolitis (NEC) occurs particularly in small babies in whom there has been a history of pre-natal or early postnatal distress leading to hypoxia. It occurs more frequently after delivery by caesarian section, and after exchange transfusion. Thrombosis of the mesenteric or intramural vessels leads first to mucosal and later to full thickness necrosis of the bowel wall. The vascular accident is thought to be secondary either to systemic hypotension or to the colonization of the bowel with endotoxin-producing bacteria. The bacteria under most suspicion are clostridium difficile and clostridium perfringens.

DIFFERENTIAL DIAGNOSIS OF X-RAY

Perforation of bowel from any other cause.

Meconium peritonitis secondary to ileal or jejunal atresia, or volvulus.

Aspiration bronchopneumonia.

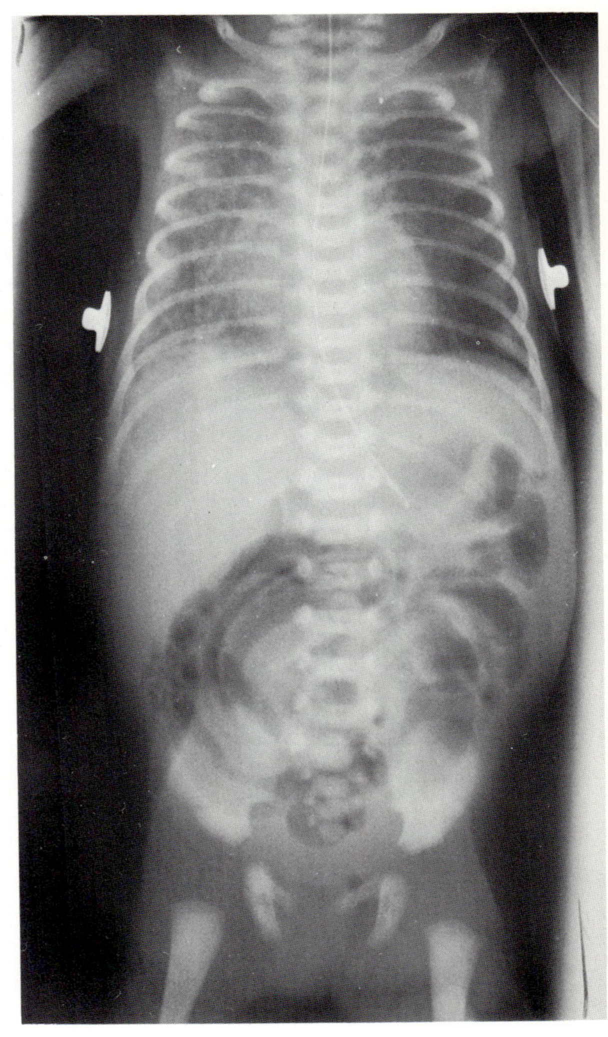

Fig. 79. Necrotising enterocolitis.

Small bowel obstruction secondary to an appendix abscess Fig. 80a and b

X-RAY APPEARANCES

Fig. 80a, supine film

Distended loops of small bowel with a 'ladder' pattern and mucosal folds characteristic of the jejunum.
Diffuse opacity of a mass in the pelvis, more marked on the right.
Displacement of the rectal gas shadow by the mass.
Opaque marker of the nasogastric tube in the upper abdomen.

Fig. 80b, erect film of same patient

Fluid levels in the dilated jejunal loops.

DIFFERENTIAL DIAGNOSIS OF X-RAY

Volvulus of the small intestine (see Fig. 71).
Paralytic ileus, when a greater number of less distended loops would be expected.
Ileo-caecal intussusception.

PRESENTATION

An abdominal illness of several days' duration with more recent onset of profuse vomiting.
Colicky pain superimposed on the previous right iliac fossa pain.
Pyrexia and anorexia.
Frequency of micturition.
Diarrhoea or constipation.
Right iliac fossa tenderness and mass.
Tenderness on rectal examination.

CLINICAL DIFFERENTIAL DIAGNOSIS

Any of the causes of mechanical obstruction of the small gut.
Pelvic abscess.

(a)

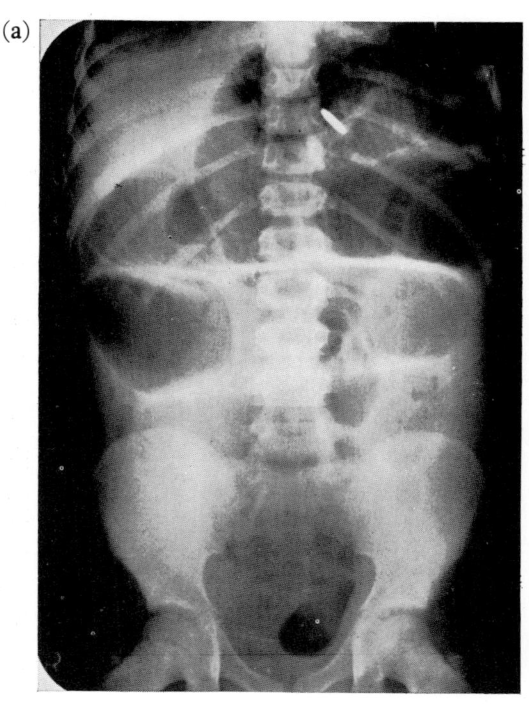

(b)

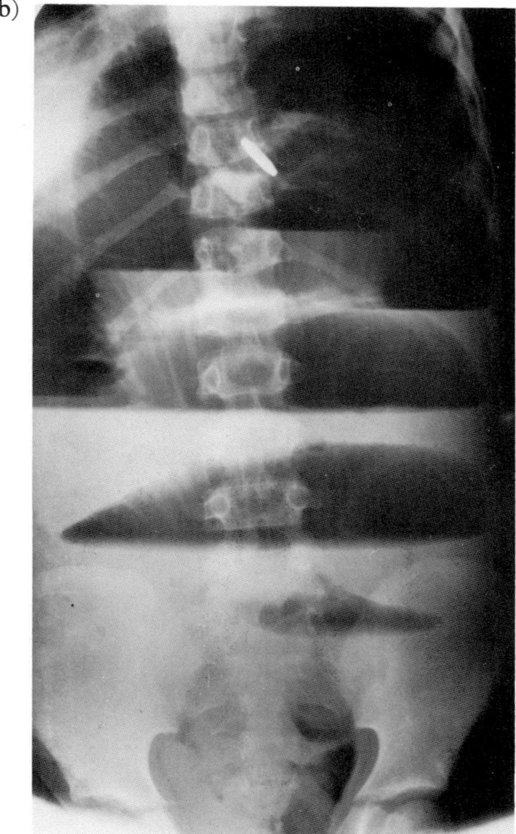

Fig. 80. Small bowel obstruction secondary to appendix abscess: **a** Supine; **b** Lateral.

Lead poisoning
Fig. 81

X-RAY APPEARANCES
(Supine film)

Small dense opacities scattered throughout the faecal content of the colon. These opacities are particles of ingested lead-containing paint.

DIFFERENTIAL DIAGNOSIS OF X-RAY

Barium residue after a meal or enema.
Bismuth mixtures taken orally for 'dyspepsia' (see Fig. 96).

In chronic lead poisoning characteristic radiological changes occur at the epiphyses.

PRESENTATION

Colicky abdominal pain, constipation, vomiting, headache.
Anaemia.
Peripheral neuritis and occasionally encephalopathy.

Lead poisoning is now rare in Great Britain, but is usually due to the child eating old lead-containing paint which flakes off toys or woodwork in the house. The ash from old car batteries which may have been burnt for heat by poor families provides another source of ingested lead.

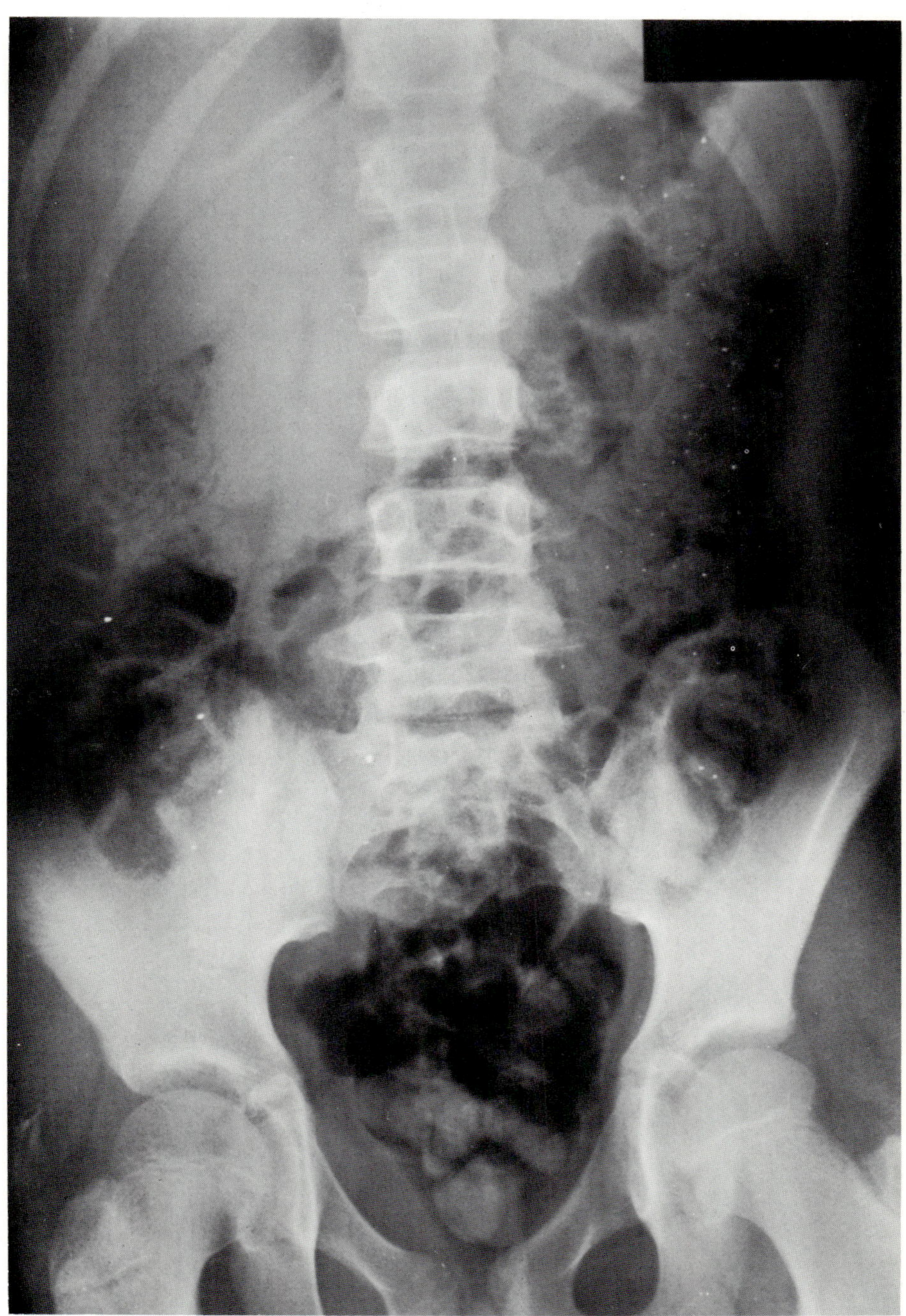

Fig. 81. Lead poisoning.

Nephroblastoma (Wilm's tumour) Fig. 82

X-RAY APPEARANCES (Supine film)

Large soft tissue mass on the left side of the abdomen.
Displacement of the gastric and the transverse and descending colonic gas shadows.
Small bowel displacement.
Absence of calcification in the mass.
Faecal masses in the rectum, sigmoid and transverse colon.
Lateral flexion of the lumbar spine, of no significance unless confirmed in an erect film.
Normal soft tissue shadow of liver.

Ultrasonography will determine whether the mass is solid or cystic. An excretory urogram is essential to identify normal function in the contralateral kidney. A late film (up to 24 hours) may give helpful information if the mass is a hydronephrotic kidney.

DIFFERENTIAL DIAGNOSIS OF X-RAY

Hydronephrosis, usually due to pelviureteric junction obstruction.
Splenomegaly.
Neuroblastoma, in which case speckled calcification in the mass may be seen.
Other retroperitoneal cyst or tumour.

PRESENTATION

Abdominal mass, sometimes noticed by the parent.
Abdominal pain, often caused by increased tension due to haemorrhage within the mass.
Haematuria.
Failure to gain weight: anorexia: pyrexia which might suggest an intra-abdominal abscess.

Abdominal palpation should be limited in order to reduce venous dissemination of the tumour.

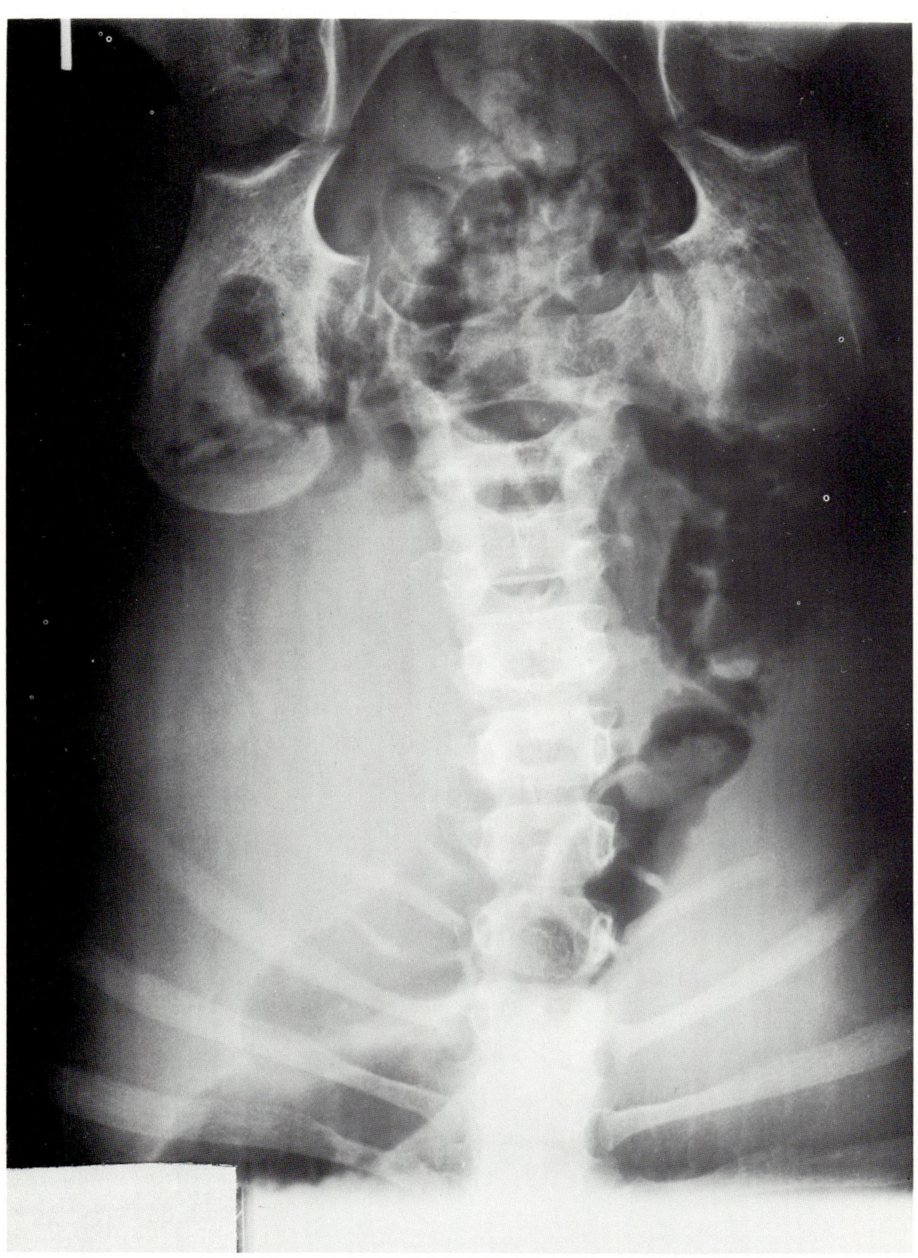

Fig. 82. Nephroblastoma (Wilm's tumour).

Hepatoblastoma
Fig. 83

X-RAY APPEARANCES
(Supine film)

Large, dense, soft tissue shadow in the upper abdomen, continuous with the liver shadow.

Normal bowel gas distribution, apart from displacement.

Splenic shadow separate from the mass.

DIFFERENTIAL DIAGNOSIS OF X-RAY

Large fluid filled stomach.

Gastric bezoar, but speckled gas shadows are invariably seen within the animal or vegetable matter constituting a bezoar.

Incisional hernia containing liver following skin cover of exomphalos or gastroschisis as an infant.

PRESENTATION

Abdominal mass noted by the parents or a doctor.

Epigastric pain or discomfort.

Failure to thrive.

CLINICAL DIFFERENTIAL DIAGNOSIS

Other hepatic tumours—either primary, e.g. lymphoma or haemangioma, or secondary, e.g. neuroblastoma.

Neuroblastoma or nephroblastoma.

Gastric bezoar.

Biliary cyst.

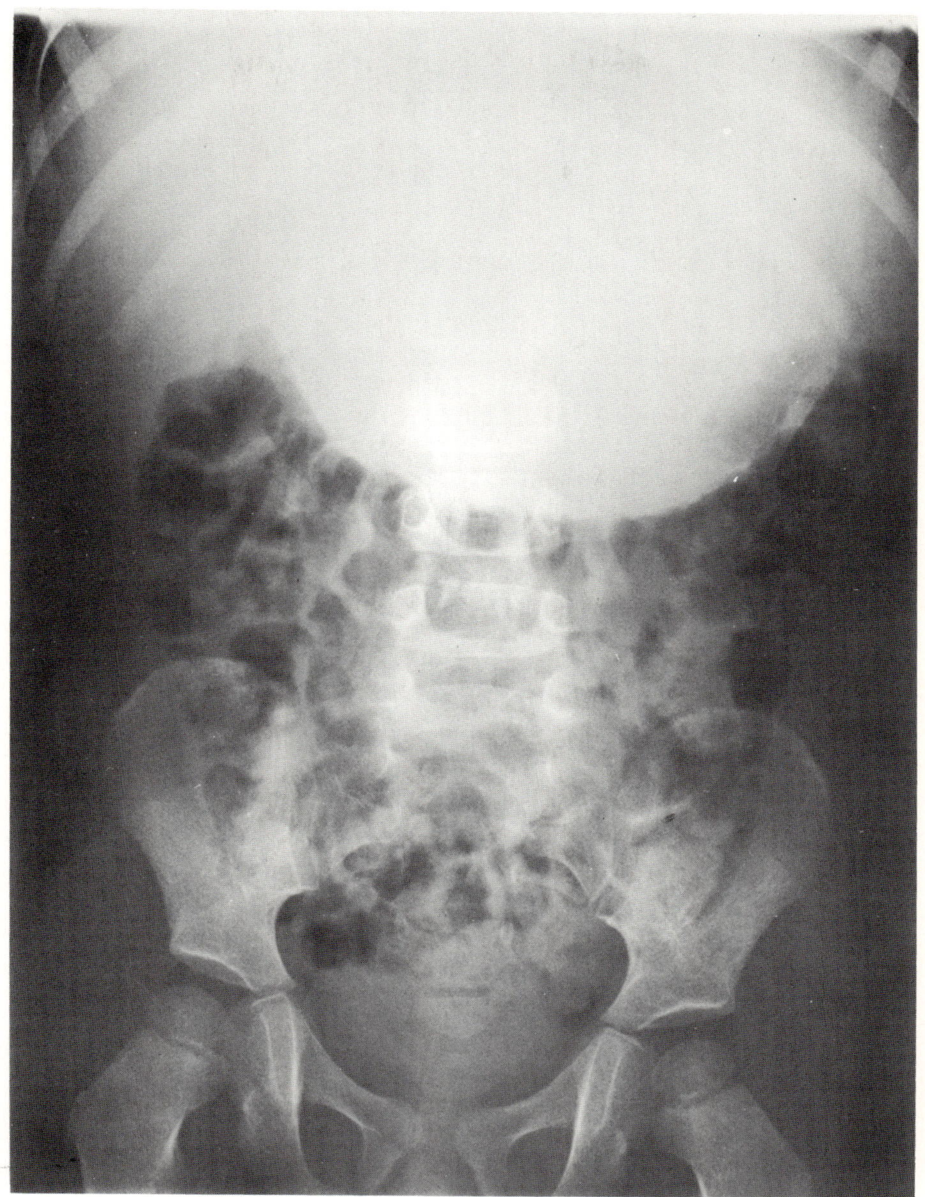

Fig. 83. Hepatoblastoma.

Chapter 6
Miscellaneous Opacities

Opacities of various types are often seen on a plain X-ray of the abdomen. They usually represent calcification of abnormal tissue, or stones occurring in the biliary or renal tracts. In spite of the conspicuous nature of many of these opacities, they may bear little relevance to the problem of acute abdominal pain.

Opacities on an X-ray may be classified as:

1 those possibly relevant to the patient's condition;

2 those which are probably incidental to the problem of abdominal pain;

3 artefacts.

Referring to the examples illustrated in this book, the first group includes:

Renal, ureteric or vesical calculi (Figs 44, 50 and 53);
Bladder calcification (Fig. 90);
Gallstones (Fig. 16);
Pancreatic calcification (Fig. 14);
Abdominal aortic aneurysm (Fig. 84);
Appendicular faecolith (Figs 21 and 22);
Bony metastases (Fig. 94);
Meconium peritonitis (Fig. 76);
Lead poisoning (Fig. 81);
Pregnancy (Fig. 58).

Examples of opacities which are probably incidental are:

Calcified mesenteric glands (Figs 24 and 95);
Phleboliths (Fig. 88);
Prostatic calcification (Fig. 88);
Adrenal calcification (Fig. 91);
Splenic artery aneurysm (Fig. 85);
Calcified cyst of the spleen (Fig. 86);
Foreign bodies within the gut (Fig. 10).

Other examples of ingested opacities are tablets and capsules which may pass through the stomach without being dissolved, or a piece of lead shot, which is not infrequently seen in the caecal region after a meal of game.

In a patient with multiple injuries some of the following may be seen on the plain X-ray taken immediately after admission:

Metal fragments, including shrapnel, bullets and shot.
Road gravel, if it contains enough lead to be radio-opaque.
Wood, which is not opaque but may be visible if covered by lead paint.

Plastic objects are usually radiolucent. Foreign bodies may be in the clothing, or in the tissues. An X-ray in another plane, with the clothing removed, will provide the answer.

Opacities in tissues may follow previous investigation or treatment. Contrast media such as Lipiodil and Myodil may persist for many years. Thorotrast, which was once widely used, was retained indefinitely in the liver and spleen and may therefore be seen occasionally in older patients, as may bismuth in the gluteal muscles of patients treated for syphilis. Tantalum gauze, sometimes used in the repair of hernias, appears as a fine dense net, while metal clips ('Liga clips'), wire sutures, orthopaedic metal prostheses and staples are easily recognizable. Separate pictures of artefacts have not been included as they vary so widely and few are typical. They may be caused by:

1 faults in the X-ray cassette;

2 marks made on the film during processing (Fig. 84);

3 intravenous drip tubing, adhesive plaster, buttons or safety-pins on the patient or the clothing.

Leaking abdominal aortic aneurysm Fig. 84

X-RAY APPEARANCES (Supine film)

Calcification outlining a large fusiform abdominal aortic aneurysm, arrowed.
Diffuse opacity of the right half of the abdomen compared with the left. In conjunction with the absent psoas shadows this suggests the presence of a retroperitoneal haematoma from posterior rupture of the aneurysm.
Duodenal gas bubble. This is probably due to local paralytic ileus caused by the retroperitoneal blood (cf. Fig. 60). More generalized ileus may develop.
Calcification of the descending thoracic aorta, arrowed.

Other unrelated features

Calcified costal cartilages.
Osteo-arthritic changes in the lumbar vertebrae.
Linear artefact on the right, probably caused during processing.

A lateral X-ray which may be taken with the patient supine will demonstrate the antero-posterior extent of the aneurysm. Sometimes this will reveal calcification which in the antero-posterior film has been obscured by the vertebrae.

DIFFERENTIAL DIAGNOSIS OF X-RAY

Calcification in a mesenteric or ovarian cyst.

PRESENTATION

Back and abdominal pain of sudden onset. Frequently there is a recent history of backache.
Signs of circulatory failure.
An abdominal mass with expansile pulsation.
Abdominal tenderness which may be localized over the mass or, when it is caused by spread of the haematoma may be separate from the mass.
Abdominal distension partly due to the mass and partly to the associated paralytic ileus.

When pain and tenderness develop in a patient known to have an aortic aneurysm the cause is usually a leak, rather than some unrelated condition.

CLINICAL DIFFERENTIAL DIAGNOSIS

Dissecting aneurysm of the aorta.
Acute pancreatitis.
Perforated peptic ulcer.
Mesenteric vascular occlusion.
Myocardial infarction.

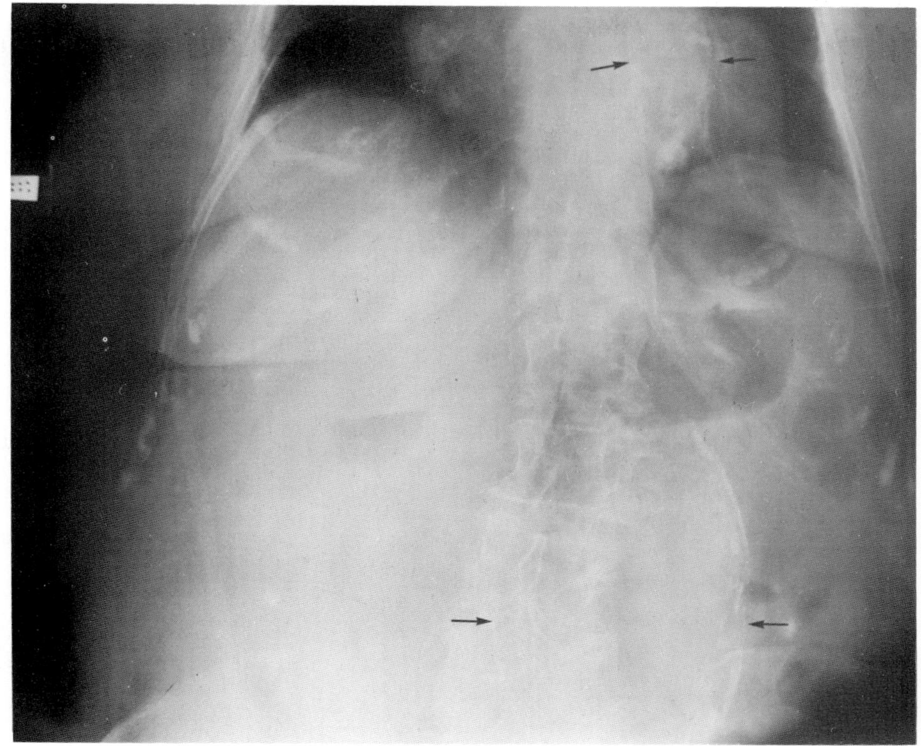

Fig. 84. Leaking abdominal aortic aneurysm.

Splenic artery aneurysm: iliac artery calcification Fig. 85

X-RAY APPEARANCES

Concentric rings of calcification within the splenic artery aneurysm in the left upper quadrant.
Calcified costal cartilages.
A dense opacity overlying the right transverse process of L.3.
Bilateral calcification of internal and external iliac arteries.

The opacity opposite L.3 may be a ureteric calculus, an ingested tablet or a densely calcified mesenteric node. Splenic artery aneurysms are uncommon, but may be multiple and may rupture. The clinical presentation is one of sudden severe abdominal pain and shock. The diagnosis most usually made is that of perforation of a peptic ulcer or, in a woman of child-bearing age, a ruptured ectopic pregnancy. A splenic artery aneurysm may rupture during the later months of pregnancy. In these younger patients calcification on a plain X-ray is less likely to be seen.

Calcified iliac arteries may be found by chance in elderly people but are often seen in patients with arterial disease who present with either lower limb ischaemia or with an abdominal aortic aneurysm. Arterial calcification may also be seen in younger patients with secondary hyperparathyroidism, e.g. in chronic renal failure.

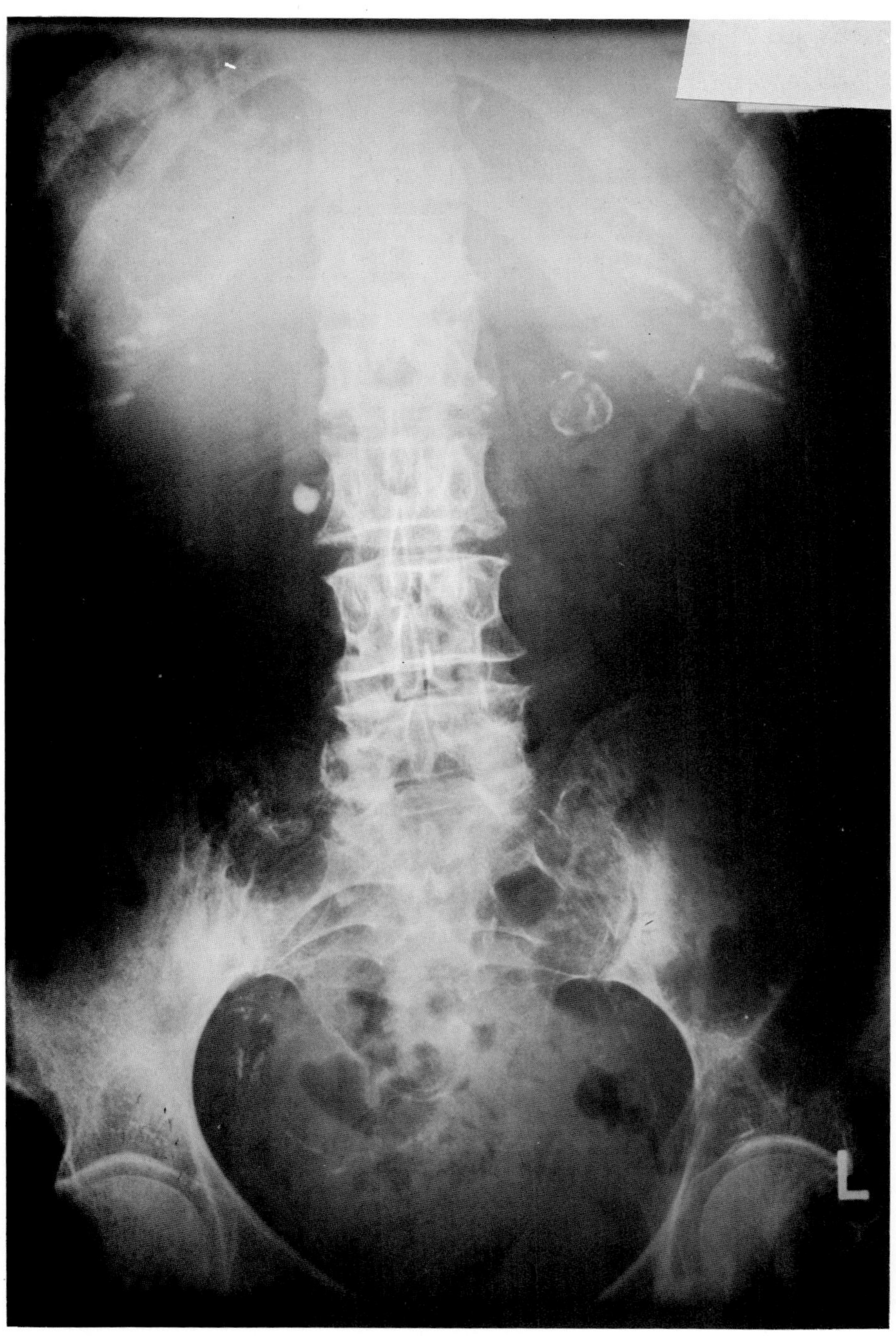

Fig. 85. Splenic artery aneurysm: iliac artery calcification.

Calcified cyst of the spleen
Fig. 86

X-RAY APPEARANCES

There is a large, calcified, smooth-walled cyst under the left diaphragm.

This proved to be a hydatid cyst of the spleen but calcification of a haemorrhagic splenic cyst produces a similar appearance. Haemorrhagic cysts are single and are a late manifestation of a spontaneous or post-traumatic subcapsular haematoma. Hydatid cysts are frequently multiple and are also found in other sites.

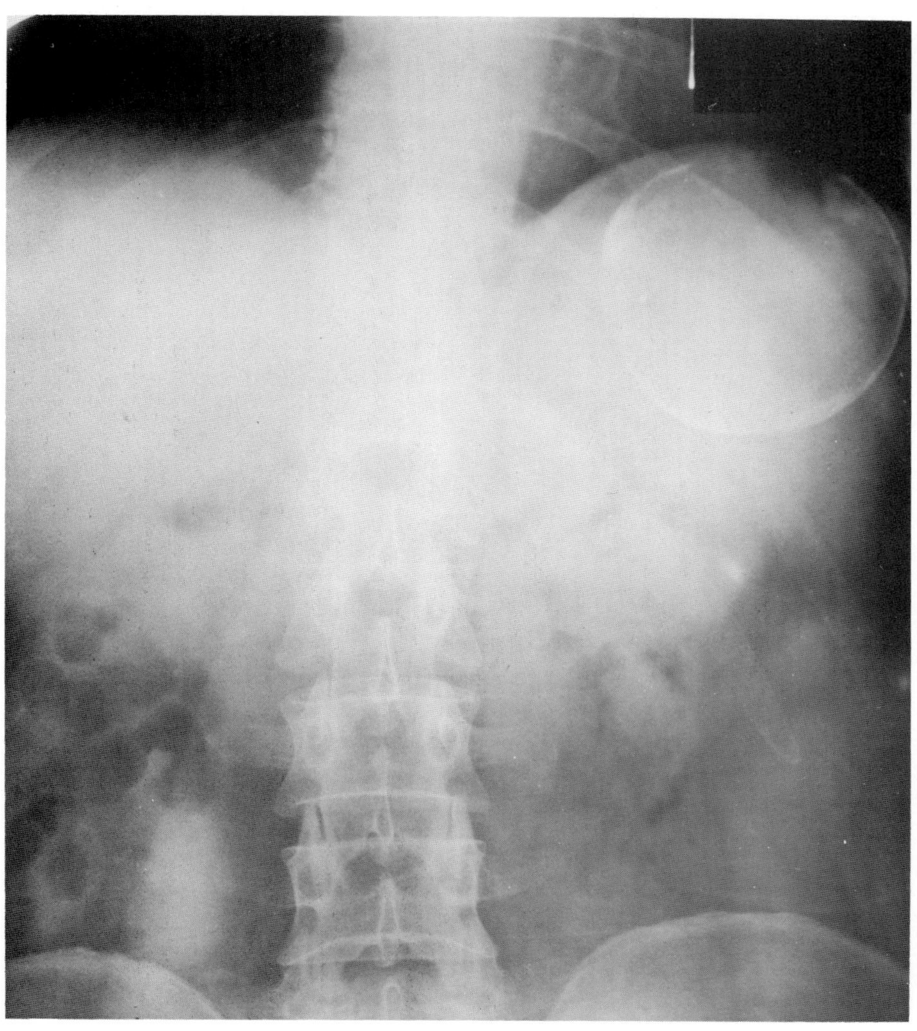

Fig. 86. Calcified cyst of spleen.

Previous lymphangiogram. Chylous ascites
Fig. 87

X-RAY APPEARANCES

The patchy opacification in the line of the iliac and para-aortic nodes is typical of a lymphangiogram. In this case there is gross abnormality of the lymphatic system, with no recognizable normal lymphatic vessels or nodes.

This study was done as part of the investigation of chylous ascites, and some of the contrast medium can be seen lying free in droplet form in the left upper quadrant.

The oily contrast medium is cleared very slowly from the lymph nodes, and may therefore persist for many months.

Note the radio-opaque marking of a shunt tube in the pelvis and left hypochondrium.

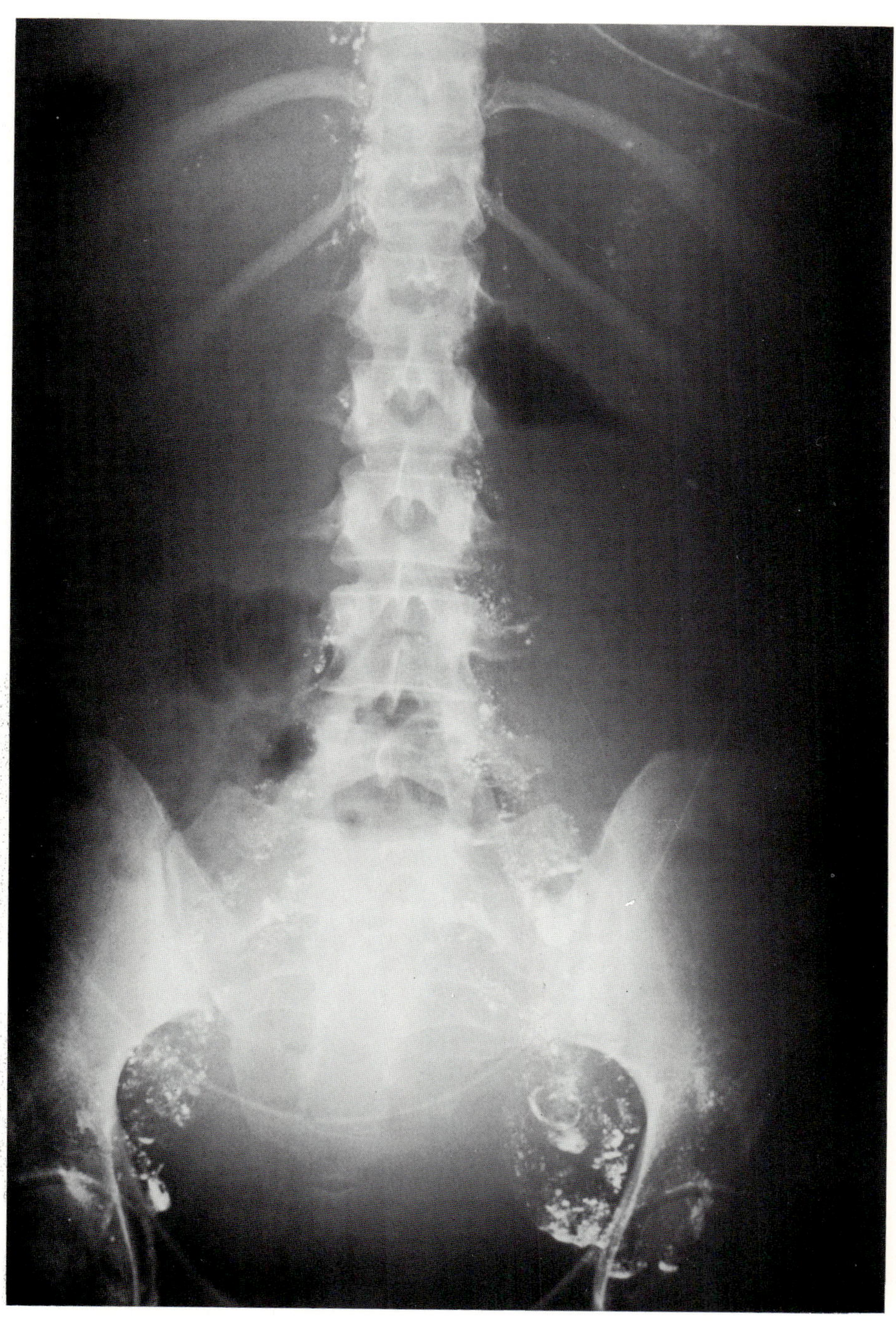

Fig. 87. Previous lymphangiogram: chylous ascites.

Prostatic calcification: phlebolith
Fig. 88

X-RAY APPEARANCES

Calcification in the region of the prostate.

The round, evenly calcified opacity just below and medial to the left ischial spine is a phlebolith.

Prostatic calcification is not uncommon. It may occur in a normal-sized or enlarged gland and the pattern of calcification is variable. Phleboliths are found in the young as well as the aged, are often multiple, occasionally have a central translucency (see Fig. 51), and occur most commonly in the veins of the pelvis, including the prostatic venous plexus. On the X-ray of a patient presenting with abdominal colic a phlebolith must be differentiated from a ureteric calculus. Phleboliths have no other significance. Prostatic calcification is similarly of no clinical significance.

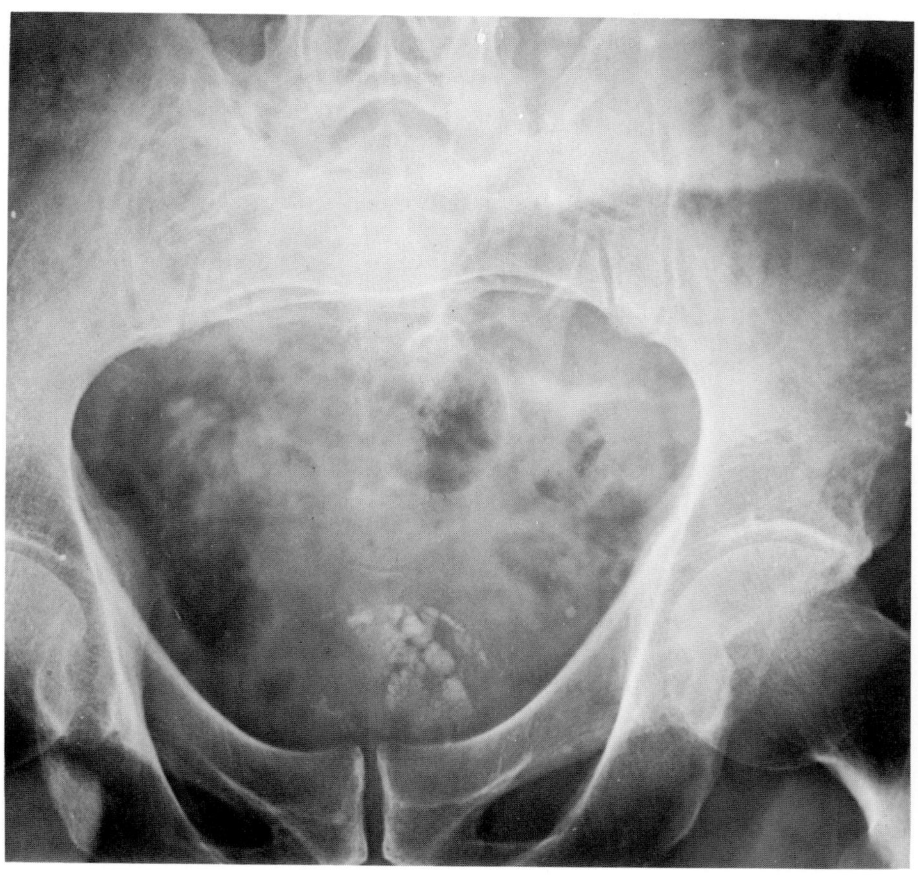

Fig. 88. Prostatic calcification and phlebolith.

Calcified uterine fibroid
Fig. 89

X-RAY APPEARANCES

Characteristic round, mottled calcification in the pelvis. Calcified fibroids may be multiple and are sometimes larger than this example. The common differential diagnosis is from calcified mesenteric lymph glands. Both conditions rarely have any clinical significance. Calcification may occur in an ovarian tumour.

There are several phleboliths in the pelvis.

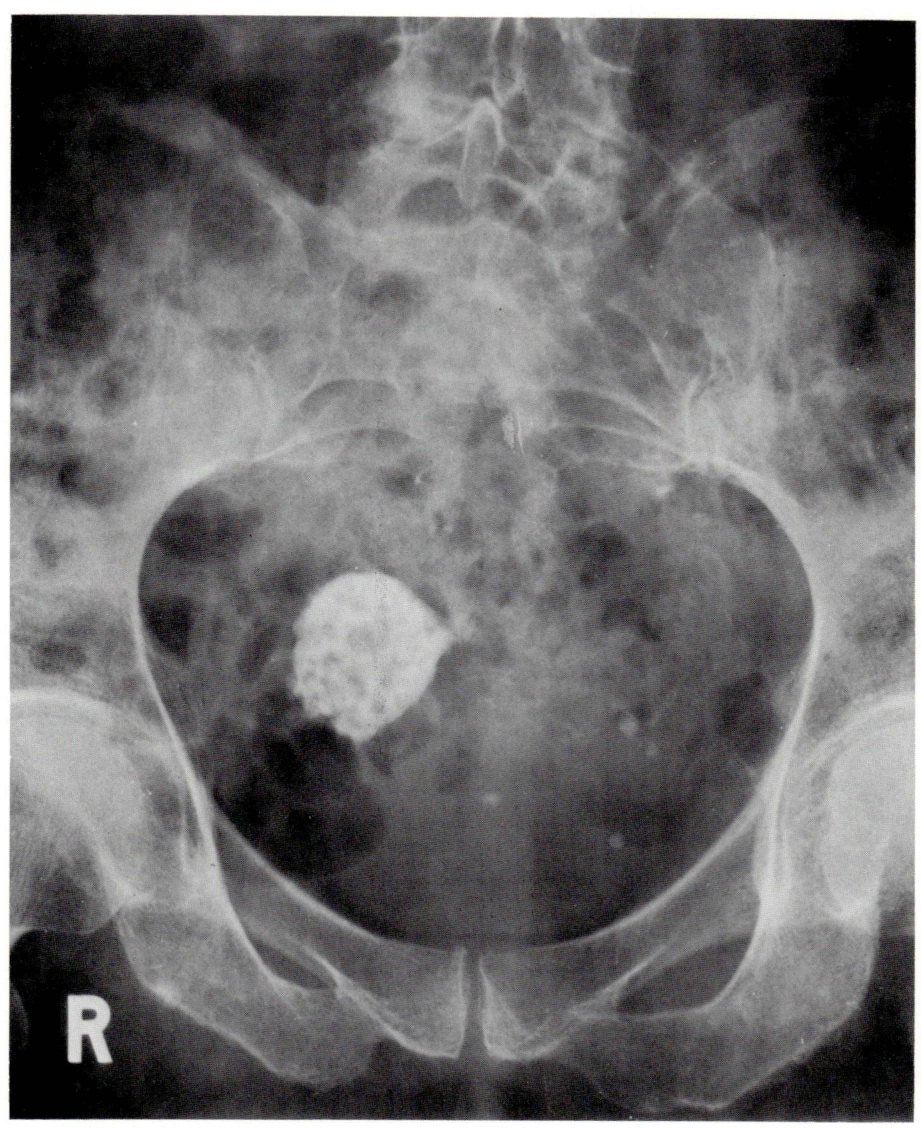

Fig. 89. Calcified uterine fibroid.

Calcification of the bladder
Fig. 90

X-RAY APPEARANCES

There is soft calcification outlining the right aspect of the dome of the bladder.
A phlebolith is present immediately above the left ischial spine (see Figs 51 and 88).

Calcification may occur in the substance of intra-abdominal neoplasms, e.g. a hepatoma or renal cell carcinoma, and neuroblastoma.

DIFFERENTIAL DIAGNOSIS OF X-RAY

Calcification in a tumour.
Calcification secondary to schistosomiasis.

Unlike tuberculous renal disease (Fig. 47), calcification following tuberculous cystitis is rare.

PRESENTATION

This patient presented with suprapubic pain due to urinary infection which was later proved to be secondary to a transitional cell carcinoma of the bladder.

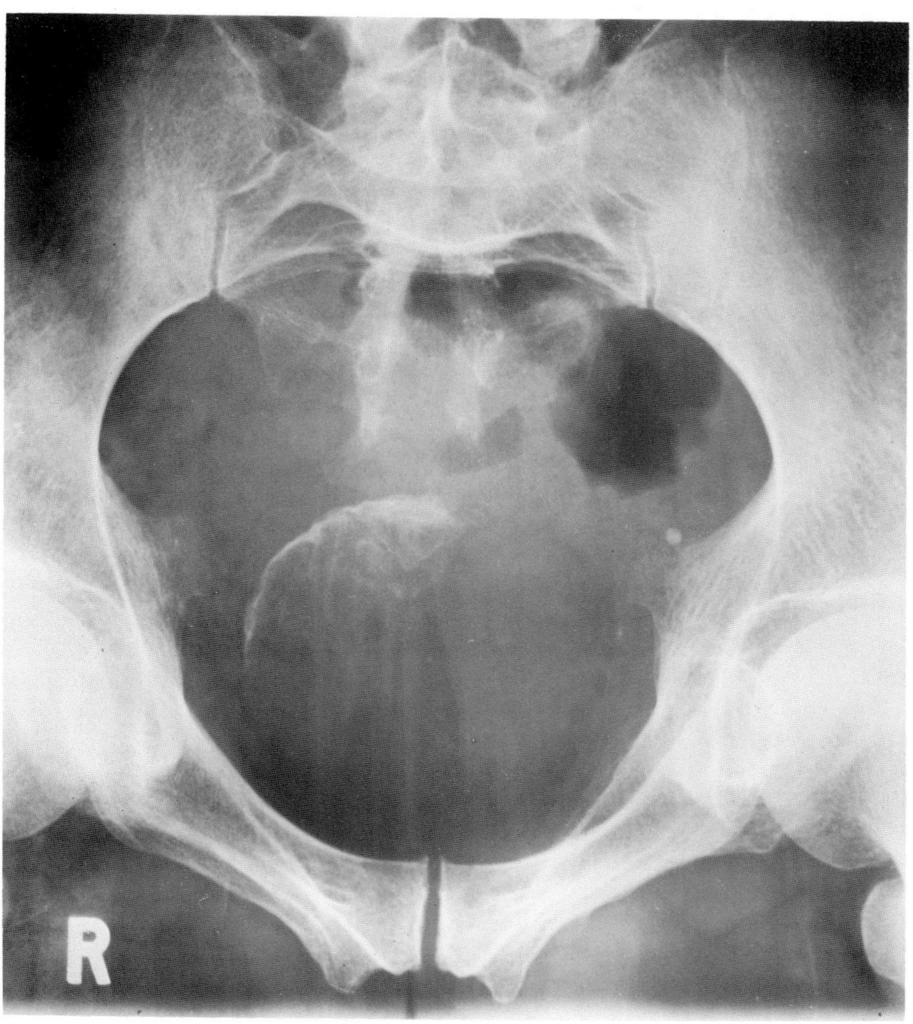

Fig. 90. Calcification in the bladder.

Adrenal calcification
Fig. 91

X-RAY APPEARANCES

This oblique film demonstrates the crescentic and mottled opacity typical of adrenal calcification.

Bilateral calcification may be seen without evidence of adrenal insufficiency but should suggest the diagnosis of Addison's disease. The other surgical implications of adrenal calcification are its association with past systemic tuberculous infection, and its differentiation from renal or hepatic calcification. Occasionally it occurs in adrenal tumours.

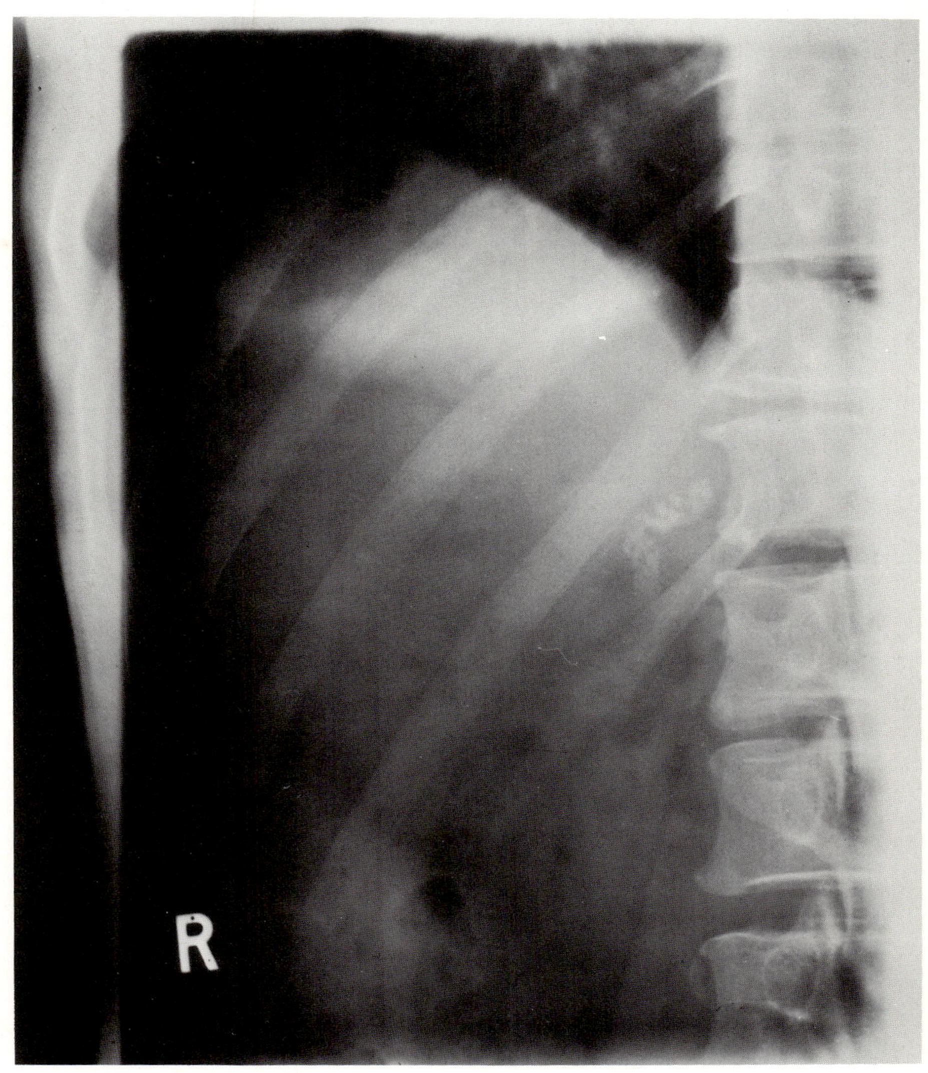

Fig. 91. Adrenal calcification.

Gall bladder calcification
Fig. 92

X-RAY APPEARANCES

'Porcelain gall bladder.'

Calcified costal cartilages are visible bilaterally, and there is generalized osteoporosis and bilateral arthritis of the hips.

Calcification in the wall of the gall-bladder is the sequel of past chronic inflammation. In the absence of localizing physical signs this X-ray appearance is unlikely to be significant.

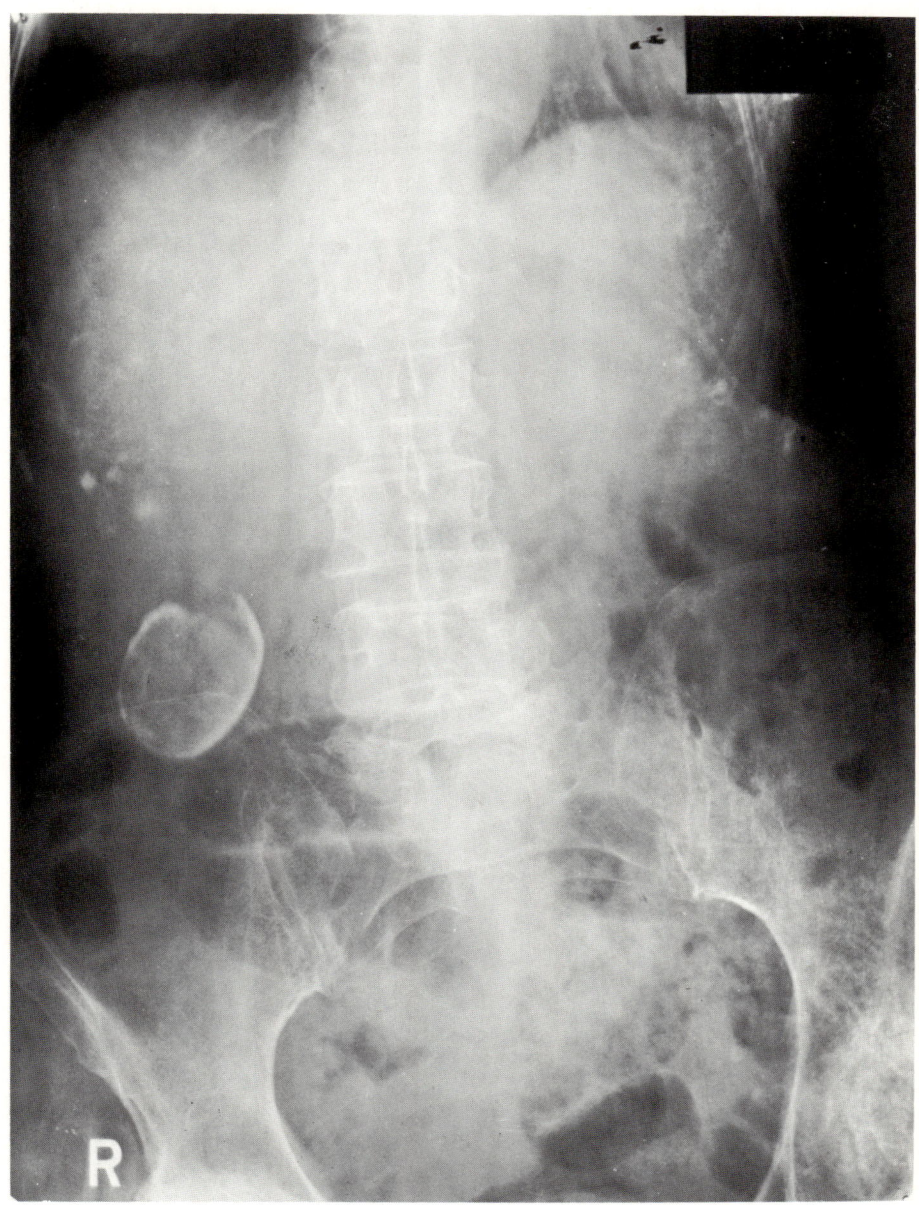

Fig. 92. Gall bladder calcification: Osteosclerotic metastases. Calcified mesenteric lymph glands.

'Limey' Bile
Fig. 93

X-RAY APPEARANCES
(Supine film)

Calcification of biliary sediment in the gall bladder. The unusual outline of the calcification is produced because this is a supine film. An erect film showed a horizontal upper margin of calcification in the fundus.

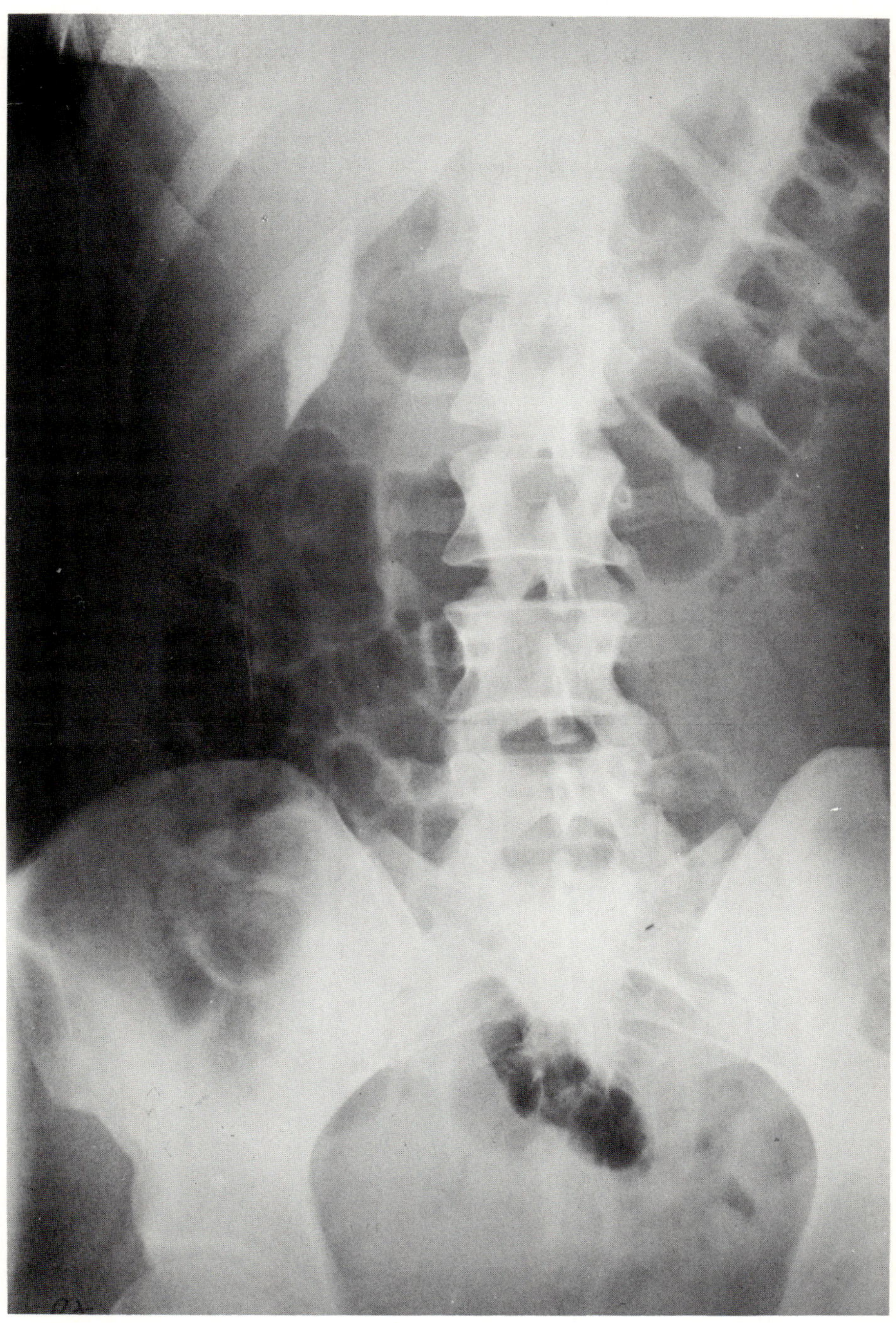

Fig. 93. 'Limey bile'.

Osteolytic metastasis: iliac bone island
Fig. 94

X-RAY APPEARANCES

The body and both rami of the right pubis show metastatic destruction of the normal bony architecture.

There is a dense 'bone island' in the right iliac bone just above the acetabulum.

Bone islands are condensations of compact bone, are not uncommon, and have no significance. They should not be confused with osteosclerotic metastases.

The soft tissue shadow of the bladder is seen within the true pelvis.

The patient proved to have a carcinoma of the prostate, causing retention of urine and producing multiple osteolytic bone metastases. Carcinoma of the prostate usually produces osteosclerotic metastases but should be considered as a cause of osteolytic metastases.

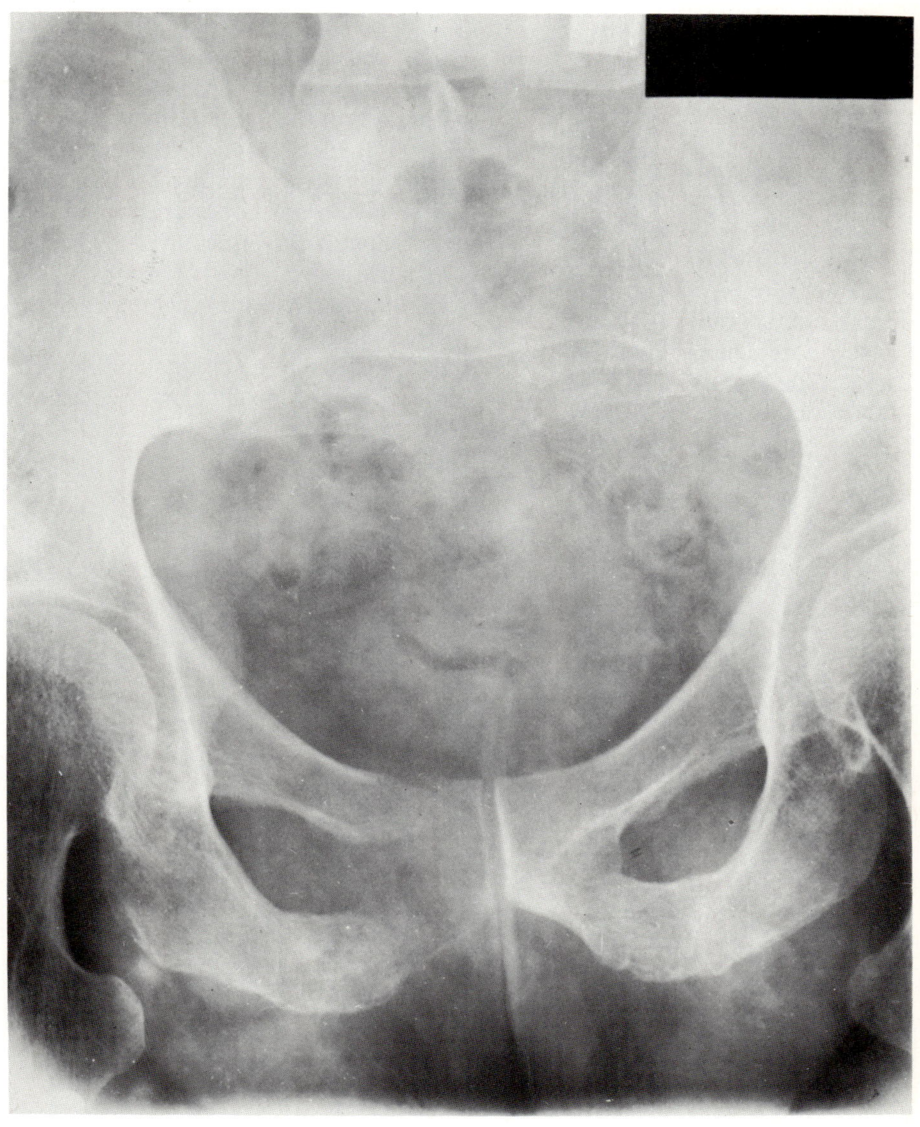

Fig. 94. Osteolytic metastasis: iliac bone island.

Renal calculus: calcified mesenteric lymph gland Fig. 95

X-RAY APPEARANCES

Homogeneous oval opacity lying just within the medial border of the right renal outline.

A similarly shaped opacity but mottled and with an irregular outline overlying the tip of the left transverse process of the fourth lumbar vertebra (in the line of the ureter).

The left renal outline is obscured by gastric and colonic contents.

The outline of the gastric fundus, arrowed.

Lateral films showed the right opacity lying posteriorly, whereas that on the left was anteriorly situated and therefore not in the ureter. An excretory urogram confirmed the presence of a calculus in the right renal pelvis, and showed normal appearance on the left.

Calcified mesenteric lymph glands usually lie in the mid or lower abdomen. They vary in size, reaching up to 6 cm in the long axis, and have well defined but irregular outlines. On subsequent films they may be seen to have moved with the patient's change of position.

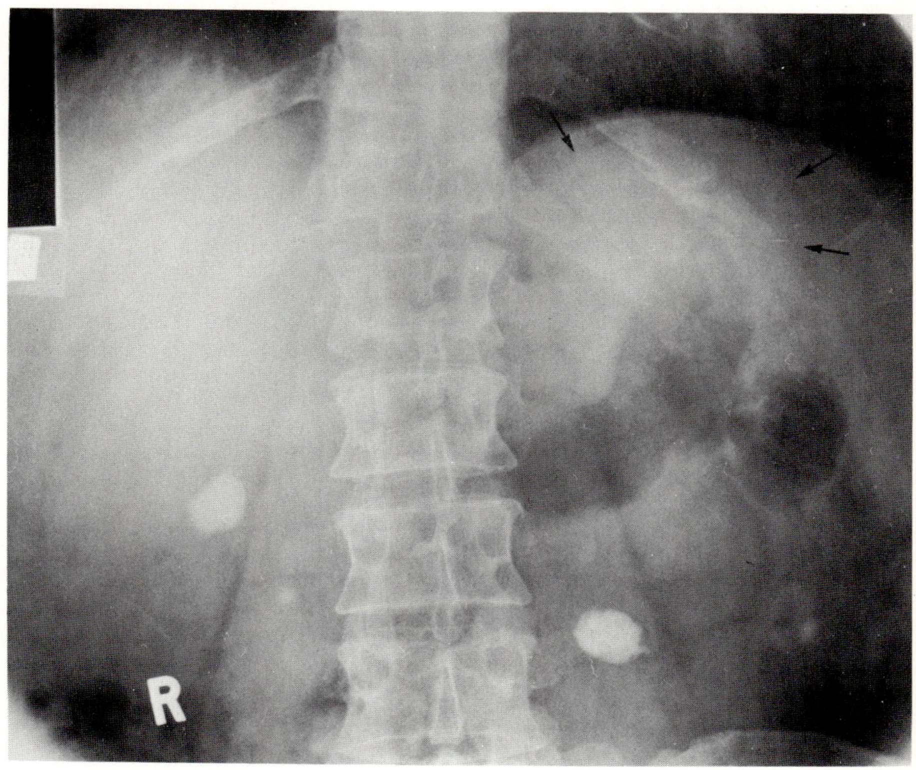

Fig. 95. Renal calculus and calcified mesenteric lymph gland.

Ingested bismuth
Fig. 96

X-RAY APPEARANCES

Speckled, dense opacities within the faecal shadows in the ascending and transverse colon.

Sacralization of the fifth lumbar transverse process.

The patient complained of abdominal discomfort for which he had been taking an antacid mixture containing bismuth. The appearances are similar to those seen after ingestion of lead particles (see Fig. 81).

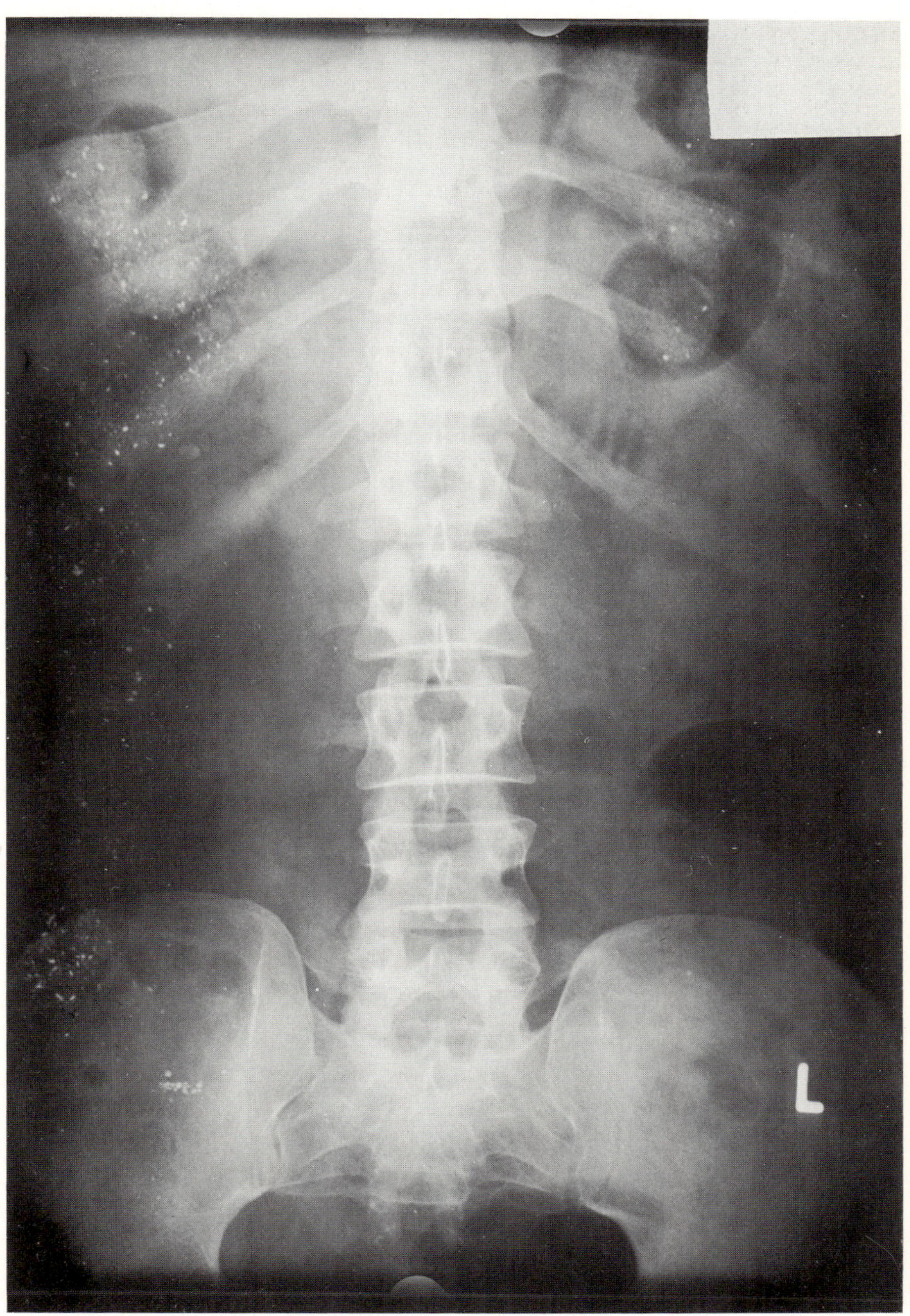

Fig. 96. Ingested bismuth.

Index

Numbers in bold type indicate pages on which principal descriptions and illustrations appear